How I Ended My Endometriosis Naturally

PRAISE FOR *HEAL ENDOMETRIOSIS NATURALLY*

"Wendy is an inspiration and so passionate about helping women with Endometriosis out of pain and achieve the success she has had herself. This book is a wonderful beginning to redirect women's journey to regaining control of their health and empower themselves to reduce their pain and suffering. Wendy's unique approach will make a positive difference in your life and in your health."

– Dr S Shutlz (MD), Lyme Ninja Radio

"Her book is well-researched and helps to address the underlying root causes of endometriosis so that you can heal yourself from a cellular level, instead of just masking the symptoms."

– Dr Anh Nguyen (PharmD), Food As Medicine

"Your book is a wonderful book. I love what you are doing and how you are helping women put Endometriosis into remission naturally. We both think differently to medical mainstream. We are carpenters so we understand reversal and let the body regenerate as our bodies are genetically programmed to be healthy."

– Dr Patrick Flynn (MD), The Wellness Clinic

"Wendy is saving the lives of women all over the world to recover from the debilitating symptoms of Endometriosis. She has been successful in helping hundreds of women overcome and heal Endometriosis. Look no further, Wendy is your go-to expert."

– Dr T J Woodham, author of The Unleashed Human

"It is marvellous the work Wendy is doing freeing women from the clutches of the Endometriosis condition and helping them conquer it naturally. You would never think Wendy had endometriosis, adenomyosis or Chronic Fatigue Syndrome by looking at her now but it is a testament to her vision that she continues sharing not only her own success but the success of the many other women she has helped be pain-free around the Globe. If you get the chance to work with Wendy she will change your body and life for good."

– Dr Tony Coope (MD)

"If you're looking for a super overview of a more natural approach to healing endometriosis, this is it. In my experience supplements can help a little but noticeable change came, exactly as Wendy says, after purging both my diet and lifestyle of all things toxic. It's a major commitment but entirely worth it – I noticed improvement in 3 days dropping wheat. Dig deep for that glimmer of belief and that you can get better, and please read this book."

– Ella, Amazon Reviewer

"I've bought many books on endometriosis over the years and this is BY FAR the best – after following the advice for nearly 2 weeks my pain nearly gone – it's like a miracle!"

– Amazon Reviewer

"This book has been a life saver! I had been suffering so much pain for so many years and I don't know why. I had tried everything to relieve them without any success… I am nearly 40 and finally getting my life back again."

– Jessica, Amazon Reviewer

"…I haven't been back to the Drs for any endo related issues since and it's purely down to Wendy sharing her incredible story. I'm pain free, lost 2.5 stone in 7 months, I'm able to enjoy life again, fully, and feel better than I have done in years. I will be eternally grateful to Wendy for writing this. Please, if you are in a similar position, PLEASE just read this book, I promise you have nothing to lose, but oh so much to gain!

– Marie West PPH, Amazon Reviewer & EndoBoss® Graduate

"This is a book worth many times it's weight in gold. In my opinion, this book and the treasure within it is a game-changer. Whilst it may appear to be for women suffering with Endometriosis please understand that it is about so much more than this. Whilst many believe that Endometriosis is incurable without significant pharmaceutical and/or surgical intervention Wendy Laidlaw shares her own journey and that of other women that she has worked with and now many more with whom she works, and demonstrates that there is another way, that that way works, and that it is a way that is open to every woman seeking to return themselves to vibrant health and vitality. But it is more than that.

In my opinion this is a book for all women and also for men seeking to find their way to wellbeing, whether supporting women with endometriosis to, and perhaps more importantly seeking to understand the core principles of vibrant health and living a fulfilled life. My lifetime in medicine, science and healing has brought home to me that every symptom and every disease has meaning, meaning that is unique to the individual. Wendy Laidlaw is a living example of this and this book an invaluable guide and inspiration that enables meaning to be found and to be used to heal and to thrive. Many, many people are already indebted to Wendy for her work. I believe countless more will continue to be grateful for generations to come."

– Dr Kim A. Jobst MA DM FRCP MFHom
Consultant Physician and Medical homoeopath
Functional Shift Consulting

Wendy Laidlaw's book takes a comprehensive look at endometriosis from a holistic viewpoint. The book is extremely insightful and well written. Women suffering from endometriosis will benefit greatly from reading this book in its entirety. I highly recommend this book to any woman who is struggling with endometriosis and desires to learn more about this topic. This book is also a valuable asset to practitioners who treat patients with endometriosis. I thought it was very useful from a holistic/ and even medical view point.

– Dr Manju Rentala MD

How I Ended My

ENDOMETRIOSIS NATURALLY

Without Painkillers, Drugs or Surgery

How I Ended My Endometriosis Naturally

OTHER BOOKS BY WENDY K LAIDLAW

Heal Endometriosis Naturally Cookbook With 101 Recipes

How I Ended My Endometriosis Naturally (available in French)

Heal Endometriosis Naturally Without Painkillers, Drugs or Surgery (available in Polish, Spanish & Swedish)

COMING OUT SOON

Endometriosis Naturally Success Stories (Part 1)

EndoBoss® 21 Day Unstoppable EndoBoss ® Challenge Workbook

Embracing Emotions, Empathy & Energy; How To Unleash Your Inner Power & Become Emotionally Empowered Naturally

Endometriosis Naturally Morning Wisdom Journal

Endometriosis Secrets; Discover The 5 Poisons Perpetuating The Condition (And How to Put It In Remission)

How I Ended My

ENDOMETRIOSIS NATURALLY

Without Painkillers, Drugs or Surgery

Wendy K Laidlaw

Founder of HealEndometriosisNaturally & EndoBoss®

How I Ended My Endometriosis Naturally

–

Copyright © 2021 Wendy K Laidlaw

For all permissions and requests, write to the author at:
support@HealEndometriosisNaturally.ZohoDesk.com

ISBN: 978-1660144624

DEDICATION

I dedicate this book to my two beautiful and incredible children, Maxine and Sebastian.

I was told on numerous occasions that I would never have these wonderful children, so their very existence should help others to see how important it is to never, ever give up hope.

Maxine and Sebastian; you both are my light, my bright joy, and my inspiration in the world. I am so incredibly proud of you both for the resourceful, passionate, and delightful young adults you have become. I love you both more than I could ever put into words, and I thank God every day for being lucky enough to have you, both as my children and in my life.

This book is also dedicated to the amazing women with endometriosis and adenomyosis who I have been called to serve, and whom I call my 'EndoBosses'.

You have made it possible for me to do work that I love and do work that is meaningful and worthwhile.

And lastly, to Ginty, my adorable chocolate Labrador, who recently passed after 16 glorious years of utter love, loyalty and companionship.

How I Ended My Endometriosis Naturally

MEDICAL DISCLAIMER

THIS BOOK IS BASED ON MY PERSONAL EXPERIENCES ONLY, SHARES MY SUCCESS STORY AND SHOULD NOT BE USED TO TAKE THE PLACE OF A MEDICAL PROFESSIONAL'S OPINION.

I am not a scientist, nor am I a medical expert on endometriosis. I am a women's health coach and consultant, who has previously suffered from endometriosis, and who has read and studied a great deal about the subject. During my recovery, I retrained in nutritional therapy, psychotherapy, and I am currently studying a psychology honours degree. However, by no means have I studied the subject of endometriosis entirely and exhaustively.

What I bring to the book is over 33 years' worth of my healing journey, my experiences, and the processes that led to my full recovery from pelvic pain and the symptoms of endometriosis and adenomyosis. What I describe is a multi-dimensional, multi-model, pragmatic approach, sharing the principles that led to my full remission using natural methods which worked well for me and changed my life.

In this updated 2nd edition, I am pleased to share that these principles have also enabled many other women with endometriosis around the world to put their condition into remission as well.

I am unable to make any claims for legal purposes and cannot promise the principles in this book will work for everyone; I can only state what worked for me.

Although these principles may not work for everyone, I dearly hope and pray that they work for you, as they did for me, so that you can be free of this chronic, debilitating condition as well. (If you get stuck or regress at any stage remember it is a sign of strength to reach out to us for further personalised support through our online programs).

The information should not be treated as a substitute for professional medical advice. What is contained within the book is only my experience.

This book is not intended to replace the medical advice of physicians or doctors. However, I would suggest you seek a medical professional who is fully supportive of your desire to consider a natural approach to the health of your body. The reader should regularly consult a physician or doctor in matters relating to her health and particularly concerning any symptoms that may require diagnosis or medical attention.

If you think you may be suffering from any other medical condition, you get a worsening of current symptoms, or have any new symptoms that are not resolving, you should seek immediate medical attention and insist your symptoms are investigated by tests that are beyond the scope of this book.

Please feel free to ask your doctor or physician to contact me to discuss any aspect of the advice suggested in the book. If you have any specific questions about any medical matter, you should consult your doctor or other professional healthcare providers.

Please use this book responsibly. You should never delay seeking medical advice, disregard medical advice, or discontinue medical treatment because of the information presented in this book.

Readers are advised to take full responsibility for their own safety and know their own limits.

The author does not take any responsibility for anybody who misuses the advice in the book.

CONTENTS

FOREWORD

Wendy describes the miserable symptoms and signs of endometriosis, moving on to the pathophysiology of such. This is vital because the road recovery is not an easy path to walk – it requires major lifestyle changes.

As a previous sufferer, Wendy has walked this path, and like so many on similar journeys, taken many wrong turns. But her experience can now lead you along the shortest and most direct route. Importantly she guides you around the terrible pitfalls which may cause irreversible damage.

The tools of the trade she employs are standard naturopathic techniques: diet, supplements, detoxification regimes, enzymes, herbals, physicals and psychologicals, all of which have a fine evidence base and are of proven benefit.

More importantly, Wendy has established the essential naturopathic tools which put recovery in the grasp of all sufferers.

She weaves these threads together to provide the tapestry and inspiration so that you can, and you must, just do it!

Wendy supplies the intellectual imperatives to give you the will to change because change you must, and change you will!

Dr Sarah Myhill Mb Bs
Author of 9 Books
'Peoples Book Prize' Winner
British Medical Association (BMA) Short-listed Author
Member of the British Society for Ecological Medicine (BSEM)

ACKNOWLEDGEMENTS

T here are so many people I want to thank for being willing

to share their ideas with me. Ideas that ultimately became the strategies and principles behind everything inside of this book.

I have learned from hundreds of people, and there are many who gave me specific ideas for this book. I have tried to give credit to original sources when possible, and apologies if I have missed anyone out. I want to mention a few of these brilliant men and women who have inspired me, in no particular order.

There are three wonderful, wise women who I want to thank, for they are all pioneers in their respective fields. These women have challenged the conventional 'medical machine' and taken the road-less-travelled in their passionate attempts to help their patients and clients. They are: Dian Shepperson Mills who is a nutritional therapist and author of the book '*Endometriosis: A Guide to Healing Through Nutrition*'; Nora Covey who helps women in the preservation of their uterus/womb through her charity Hysterectomy Education Resources and Services (HERS), and her book '*The 'H' Word*'; and Dr Sarah Myhill who has authored many books and who also helped me so passionately and with such dedication to recover from chronic fatigue syndrome (CFS) and mitochondria dysfunction. Thank you to you all for your unwavering faith in me, delightful strength of character, and for holding the torch to lead the way for my recovery through many dark times.

I also wish to thank Suzy Grieve, editor of Psychologies Magazine, who first introduced me to the concept of life coaching and another way of living my life through her 'The Big Leap' program; Jess Thompson from The Ultimate Health Clinic in London; Lion Goodman for his unique, innovative and excellent support in 'The Belief Closet' program; Dr Tony Coope for his kindness and patience; and Julia Cameron for her book 'The Artist Way'. They have all been instrumental in my recovery and I thank them for their patience and kindness when I felt lost.

I want to thank Pam Williamson, my counsellor and EMDR therapist, who has helped me to navigate the journey over the past few years. Her professionalism, reliability, consistency, and patience have been invaluable as she guided me through some emotionally turbulent times. Pam's unwavering support and belief in me have given me the ability to write this book and make this process available to other women around the world.

I also wish to thank Russell Brunson for writing his incredible marketing books and sharing his own journey. The creation of his online marketing programs has provided me with the encouragement and direction to self-publish and promote my book along with my online programs. It was his pathways that provided me with the steps so I could share my success story with you now.

I want to thank my friend and business coach, Christian Fioravanti, who was integral in believing in me and my mission right from the beginning of my online journey. When I felt like giving up at times or was frightened of my next step, he was always there to encourage me. I could not have got this far without his incredible energy, passion and generosity of spirit.

I would also like to thank my friend and business coach, Vince Green, for being so generous with his time, insight, and commitment in helping me share my message to women with endometriosis.

I want to thank my dear friend and business coach, Sarah Morrison, for her love, her kindness and support over the past few years. It is lovely to work with an incredible woman who has such heart and strength, plus softness and integrity all rolled into one.

And, last but by no means least, I wish to thank Maxine I. K. Anderson and Sebastian C. N. Anderson, my darling children, who have been incredible throughout the past five years in particular. Their wisdom, love and encouraging belief in me when this journey got tough has been enlightening and so uplifting – and I feel so blessed. Their work ethic and contribution to this book is endless. The hours, days, weeks and months that we all pored over this book together has enabled this updated version to be printed again now. I thank them both with all of my heart.

None of this would have been possible without all the people I've mentioned above. Thank you to all of you who have helped me to share my endometriosis success story and message to millions.

A MESSAGE FROM THE AUTHOR

T his whole book is a message from me, the author, of course, but as I update my original version that was printed in 2015, I am more excited than ever to share the contents of this book.

Firstly, you may have noticed that the title of the book has been amended slightly from the first edition, to prevent any confusion about the contents and purpose of this book. As such, it will be more apparent to readers that this book reflects my own success story and journey along with a step by step guide of what worked for me.

I have amended and updated some areas of the book, plus added in some extra chapters to demonstrate some of my new understanding. However, I will cover in even more depth the areas that affect our body and emotions in my upcoming book *Embracing Emotions, Empathy and Energy*.

I look back to 2015, and I feel I have grown even more, with a broader knowledge and understanding of what it takes to be a happy and healthy human: physically, emotionally and spiritually. I braved the fear of the trolls, toads, and toxic people to reveal a stage of my life and journey that was incredibly tough, yet also empowered me in ways that I never knew were possible.

The more I learn, I realise, the less I know, and therefore I am continually hungry to keep educating myself and others of the marvellous power we have over our body, mind, and spirit.

So here I am, revisiting this labour of love with the hope and intention of you, the reader, being inspired to follow my pathway and become pain-free too.

I am still sitting with my pain-free body after putting my Stage IV endometriosis and adenomyosis into remission, and reflecting and poring over the words I wrote almost five years ago.

When it came time to revisit and go through this original book, I initially crossed things out and added bits in and so on. But then I realised something quite profound.

I have changed and continued to grow since I first wrote my original book. It was almost a different Wendy that was editing the original book, and it did not feel right to make some of the changes I wanted to make, because a part of me thought I might be reducing the quality of the text and who I was at that time of writing it.

You see, I wrote the first edition with the particular energy of haste and hurry, wanting this vital information out to as many women as possible. I was up early in the mornings, and working until late into the evenings. I was not able to type the words fast enough to keep up with all the thoughts that were streaming into my head, and all I wanted to share.

All I knew was that I need to get this information written down, published and out quickly, to give other women hope and a pathway.

I wanted women to feel and sample this new sense of freedom I had then, and still have now. I never wanted any woman to suffer in the way I had, or for as long as I had.

I do admit to being somewhat petrified the first time I pressed that all-important '*publish*' button. Once done, I bolted for cover under the duvet and stayed there, in fear of the trolls, for a few hours. It was/is a truly terrifying experience to lay yourself bare on paper this way, with all of your thoughts and feelings and experiences laid out into the public domain, in print, for the world to read: and of course, to judge.

Yet, I know I had been full of utter despair at points on my journey. There were times I was literally on my knees praying for all of the endometriosis answers to be in one place and in one book, so that I could take back control of my body and life. My whole intention was to share all that had worked for me, so that women did not have to spend months or years trying to figure it all out on their own as I did.

The months and years of my study, research, trial and error that I had documented and journalled as I battled endometriosis for 33 years, all came together to form parts of this book. So, this was why I felt propelled to share my success as soon as possible.

"*Feel the fear and do it anyway,*" they say – and that is what I did for this book.

Sadly, in the midst of my endometriosis journey, I had come to believe that this physical and emotional suffering was ordinary for me. Back then, I had resigned myself to the fact that this was how my life was meant to be – that I was supposed to suffer. That I was being punished for some unknown crime. That I was destined to have a life full of pain – physically, mentally, and emotionally. Because that was all I had ever known.

I never thought in a million years, when I started this new pathway and journey, that I would have the freedom from pain and suffering that I have now.

Healing endometriosis was not an easy journey, and it takes time, of course, to see results. But I promise you – it is worth it to be pain-free. So, once you start this new journey, keep going. It is so worth it to get to the destination. The secret to the success of this journey is to make a firm, dedicated commitment to put yourself first and let no one stop you from getting the life you seek.

Once you start on your new pathway and follow the suggestions in this book, positive signs will start to become evident in your glorious body – your body that is always trying to heal itself.

And yes, it is entirely natural to doubt if this new pathway will work!

Yes, it is entirely natural to think, *"Will I be the one it does not work for?"*

And yes, it is entirely natural to have down days, sad days, flare days and bad days where you may feel like giving up.

But just take one day at a time.

For the occasional women who may struggle to get consistent results, or who hit a block on this new recovery journey, please remember that healing takes time. Reach out to us for online support if you need it. We are all guilty of being super-impatient these days. So be realistic with the time frames for expected results. Allow at least six months for noticeable results, and anywhere between 9 and 12 months for long-lasting change.

This incredible body of yours ALWAYS wants to heal itself and this book will ask you to become a detective to figure out what may be preventing your own body from healing naturally.

This journey may stretch you and challenge your faith at times but remember that asking for support is not a sign of weakness – far from it. It takes great courage to reach out for help from safe women and the right women who have walked the path successfully ahead of you.

Some women may also need more personalised emotional support and coaching due to unresolved traumas or childhood mistreatment, and I am pleased to share that we have created more tailored online programs designed to help with that aspect too.

However, a word of warning; watch out for the naysayers.

Beware of the toxic and negative people who may feel threatened by your desire to take a new pathway. You will need to learn to protect yourself from them. Surround yourself with people who appreciate you, build you up, make you feel good about yourself and who truly believe in you.

I call them 'Believing Mirrors' – people who reflect your inner greatness and strength back to you.

If you cannot find supportive women, then consider joining our safe and loving community. Learn how to become an EndoBoss® and be amongst other EndoBosses who, like you, are taking back power and control of their body one day at a time.

Or consider joining our 21 Day Challenge, where you can put a pinky toe into the water of what it is like to meet other sensitive and wonderful women like you.

Nelson Mandela said it eloquently, *"It always seems impossible until it is done."*

And this is so, so true.

Yet, every month I am witness to more and more women coming through my online programs, defying medicine and putting their endometriosis, adenomyosis, cysts and fibroids (along with other conditions) into remission, all naturally. It is so joyful to watch the EndoBoss® journey!

Equally, every few months, I hear from EndoBoss® Alumni, who were previously told they would never fall pregnant, and/or who thought they were infertile – then email me to share their joyous news of pregnancy. So far, we have had 19 babies from 17 women going through our programs and we hope that these figures will keep growing.

If this book helps you to live the joyful life you were destined to live, then all this work will have been a success.

I heard an interesting story the other day. It is the story of two little mice that I thought it apt to share.

There were two little mice who both fell into a bucket of cream.

The first mouse quickly gave up and disappeared down deep into the liquid.

But the second mouse made a firm resolve and commitment to herself that she would not quit.

She had no choice.

She had to do something different, and giving up was not an option.

The second mouse was determined.

She persevered, and she struggled so hard that eventually – you know what? She churned that cream so thick that it turned into butter, and she stepped up and out and jumped about with glee.

As of this moment, I am that second mouse!

You deserve to be pain-free and living a life of joy and freedom, and I hope you will join me and all the other women around the globe who, with help and guidance, have achieved the same results of becoming an EndoBoss®.

It has been delightful to receive regular emails from those women who have been helped by my book. Women who have shared how their body has responded slowly, but surely, to my suggestions and how, over time, their pain has reduced and then been eliminated.

So, thank you to those who email me to share their successes. It warms my heart and keeps me going. Your emails and success stories help to inspire me to put myself out publicly onto the internet and keep sharing this message of hope with more women around the globe.

Nonetheless, I hope that this book continues to pave the way for you and gives light towards the pain-free life that you deserve to live.

Benjamin Franklin said there are three types of people in the world: Immovables, Moveables, Movers. Which type of woman are you? I already know you are a Mover because you are reading this book.

Make sure to become an even bigger 'Mover' and an EndoBoss® by taking the small, daily actionable steps every single day.

It has taken great leaps of courage and growth for me to put myself forward and share this journey with you in this way. My sole aim (or my soul's aim!) was to step out of my comfort zone and share this knowledge in the hope that it might help at least one woman.

I am pleased to share that helping one woman has now turned into helping thousands of women around the globe and so I feel that what I went through was not in vain.

As the Tanzanian Proverb says, "*Little by little, a little becomes a lot*".

Please do email us and share your journey and success, and you may be lucky enough to be featured in our next paperback edition of *Endometriosis Success Stories* by emailing: Support@HealEndometrisoisNaturally.ZohoDesk.com.

Finally, I want to say that I have so much admiration for you for starting this new journey!

I hope you enjoy this updated edition and I cannot wait for you to join me, and all of the other Alumni, to become a boss of your endometriosis – an EndoBoss®!

To your health!

Wendy

Introduction

* * *

The definition of insanity is doing the same thing over and over and expecting different results

— Albert Einstein

T he pain of endometriosis is a unique and chronic experience. The pain can be dragging, scraping, and pulling. It will often feel like barbed wire rubbing up and down your insides. The occurrence of pain can happen every few weeks or days. For some, the pain will not lessen at all during their endometriosis experience.

You may go to the doctor, but many doctors will not understand the condition right away, if ever. Some will make you feel as if you are making it up, by insinuating that you are somehow imagining it. Some might label you as 'neurotic'. Some will give you birth control pills, painkillers or prescribe surgery. But the pain is there and no matter what they suggest, it still lingers.

You may feel depressed, lost, and alone. You just want to get on and live your life, but you are tired. The constant pain has weakened your body, and it feels as if the disease is dragging you down.

You may have thought that once you got a diagnosis, all would become better for you. You may even have had surgery to get a diagnosis, and had hoped that the surgery would be the 'cure'. You may have become worse after the surgery and then sought another operation, then another, and another.

However, operations in the abdominal area almost always cause adhesions (areas of scar tissue similar to the white skin on top of a chicken breast), which attach themselves to other organs, pulling and dragging them and sometimes tying them in knots. Adhesions are only one of the many complications and side effects that can come as a result of surgery.

The millions of women who have endometriosis know how utterly debilitating it is. The unexpected nature of this invisible disease makes it difficult to prepare or plan from one month to the next. The pain can make you double up in an instant or send you to bed for two to three days on end. You try to explain the widely varying array of pain to friends, family, or work colleagues, but they will never understand unless they have endometriosis themselves. How can they? On the outside, you 'look okay', even if your insides are screaming in agony. Having endometriosis can cause you to feel lonely. You just put up with the pain and hug the hot water bottle tighter, with the hot water bottle becoming your best friend.

Ten years ago, research suggested, terrifyingly, that around one in ten women of reproductive age (that is between the ages of 15 and 49) suffered from endometriosis. Let us look at it this way – that was around 176 million women worldwide experiencing the condition.[1] Today, in 2020, up-to-date research shows similar figures or, in other words, no improvement.[2] Now, that is a lot of women suffering needlessly.

What concerns me most of all, as someone who suffered extensively for over 33 years, is the lack of information about the alternative options available to women. Although the invention of social media on the internet – such as health forums, Twitter, and Facebook – has allowed more women to come together to share their pain, despair, and to feel less alone, those above figures show that globally, endometriosis is not getting any better. This is in spite of the efforts of modern medicine.

The medical profession relies heavily on the pharmaceutical and surgical routes when they process women with this disease, but they do not address the underlying causes. Doctors prescribe women pills that are full of chemicals, or cut them open in surgery and damage them for life. Very few medical practitioners ever fully explain the real horrors and long-term side effects of the 'gold standard' procedures offered to women.

The emergence of charities like Hysterectomy Education Resources and Services (HERS) and The She Trust saved me from a lot of heartaches, and the information they provided allowed me to retain my uterus. Sadly, these organisations are in the minority, and a lot more needs to be done to educate all women, especially young girls upon commencement of menstruation, that period pains are not 'normal'. Young girls need to learn how to empower themselves to identify the root causes of inflammation before endometriosis becomes a problem for them. Prevention is far better than a 'cure'.

This book will explore the factors that I found inflamed my endometriosis. This includes the compounding effect of many poisons, dioxins, toxins, plastics, parabens, pesticides, chemicals, poor diet, and poor nutrition which – when combined – can cause severe hormone imbalances. Also, our impatient society with the 'better, faster, more, now' attitude only serves to increase stress, and intensify the pain that is uniquely endometriosis. It will also explain the genetic component, which is widely recognised by the medical profession as a significant cause of endometriosis.

This book will dispel the beliefs of, "*there is no other option*", "*I have to take pharmaceutical drugs*", "*I have to get a surgical diagnosis*" and "*I have to have another operation*". These statements often trap many women in the 'Medical Machine' and it prevents them from taking back power and control. It stops them from taking things into their own hands. This book will help demystify the natural process of healing and putting diseases into remission, by explaining how the body works, and how even a small change can make a big difference. It will tackle your self-doubts, concerns, and worries about time, money, and feeling alone.

The book will take a step-by-step approach that will enable you to understand and do all of the following:

- Start on your own path by learning how to approach endometriosis naturally

- Break the barriers that are preventing you from owning your power

- Learn that it is never too late to walk away from the medical machine

- Then use your new knowledge to help other women with endometriosis stop their pain

We often ask why only one woman in a family of four sisters develops the condition, and not the others. What are the predisposing factors that affect some women and make them more at risk of developing the condition? The reason is in the interaction between genes and environmental stressors. It is widely acknowledged nowadays that the cause of many diseases and conditions is not just either having the genetic predisposition to it, or experiencing stressors in our environment, but in the interaction of both.

What this means is that an individual may have a genetic vulnerability to developing a condition, but for them to develop it, they need to experience environmental stressors so that the gene/genes can be expressed. Whilst this is not the case for all conditions, environmental stressors do mostly appear to cause – or at least increase the severity of – many diseases, including endometriosis. So, even if your grandmother, mother, or older sister has endometriosis, it does not mean that you will have to suffer too. Throughout this book, the multiple environmental stressors that can lead to the onset of endometriosis will be covered. By addressing these, you may be able to prevent or reverse your endometriosis.

Endometriosis is an estrogen-dominant condition believed to be caused and triggered by a combination of different aspects – genetics, environment, retrograde menstruation, dioxins, embryonic cell growth, issues within the immune system and the spreading of endothelium cells through the bloodstream or lymphatic system. Many of these will be explained later on in the book.

This book tries to address those various aspects through a multi-layer approach and principles. Like peeling back the layers of an onion, you will be uncovering and attempting to identify what the triggers are for you. Once identified, then the book will show you how to eliminate them, or swap them out with natural alternatives. Where modern medicine and many alternative therapies fail is by falling into the trap of claiming a condition has arisen from a single cause that applies to everyone. However, by reading this book and addressing endometriosis naturally, you will learn an integrative approach and develop a holistic view of your whole person.

The principle behind this book is to guide you gently, slowly and consistently out of the medical machine – the maze that is pharmaceuticals, drugs, and surgery – and introduce you to the wonder that is your body. The body is ALWAYS wanting to repair and regenerate itself, and by allowing it to do so, you will, ultimately, achieve a pain-free body.

The book will also look at my journey of suffering and recovery. It details how I found a natural way out after over three decades of living with a condition that prevented me from planning – or living – a normal life. It details the approach that ended my endometriosis pelvic appendicitis-like pain, the heavy flows, the clots, the cramps, the bloating, and suffering I experienced. I will explain how I achieved this without the involvement of any medical practices or drugs.

I reached my symptom-free goal with my uterus intact through understanding the premise that the body always wants to repair and regenerate itself naturally, and that this has to be our starting position. Then I learned how to peel back, slowly, the layers of my body, my brain, and my life to be able to uncover the what, why, how, and who behind my pain and the reason why my body was not healing.

It was not an easy journey, but it has changed my life. I am far better today than I have ever been.

I look forward to you joining me on a new journey – on the right path, and with a roadmap in your hand – to addressing how to approach your body's incredible ability to regenerate and repair naturally.

Now, let us begin…

Chapter 1 -

A Woman With Endometriosis – Why Me?

* * *

We are what we repeatedly do. Excellence, then, is not an act, but a habit

– Aristotle

I could barely pronounce its name when I first became aware of

endometriosis (which is pronounced as en-doe-mee-tree-O-sis), but I certainly knew its symptoms. I had my first monthly cycle at age 11, and it was awful. Unlike all my school friends, right from the beginning I was in endless pain every month. Back then, I felt like I was the only one who suffered terribly. None of my friends seemed to be as troubled as I was, or have the chronic cramps I had. Their periods would come and go without a hitch. From that point on, I strived hard to ignore the pain. I even used the 'mind over matter', positive thinking mindset to try and will the pain away, and pretend all was okay every month. I was also too scared to ask anyone for help, for fear of embarrassment and looks of disdain.

For the next 30 years, I would come to dread my period arriving every month. The initiation into adulthood was so embarrassing, with the crippling period pains which ensued without abatement month in, month out, year after year. Barbed wire scraping, acute appendicitis-like throbbing, beating, pounding, pulsing, flashing, shooting, jumping, sharp, cutting, lacerating, gnawing, wrenching, pulling, searing, tingling, sickening, suffocating, gruelling, agonising, torturing, and piercing are just some of the words that can be used to describe the pain. It was like an endless endurance test. An endurance test that I felt I was losing every month. I came to dread anyone asking me how I was. I would pretend and say, "I am fine", for fear that telling them the truth would sound like I was feeling sorry for myself.

The dragging sensations in my pelvis would travel down my legs, around my lower back, and the headaches would turn into migraines. I was always tired, exhausted, and out of energy. I kept myself going by pumping up on sugar, which I grazed on all day. That was the only way I could function properly, and I needed it – I needed it because, at the age of 40, I was not only fighting the pain of endometriosis but running a full-time business, looking after my family, and keeping my house in order.

I would always experience heavy flow and flooding of dark red, thick blood clots every period. Oh, the flooding scared me when I was young – I always thought I was dying. I used to wonder how you could lose so much blood in a day and still live. It would literally pour out of me, leaving me drained, weak, and utterly exhausted. Not surprisingly, the heavy flow caused me to have an aversion to wearing white or light-coloured trousers. The sanitary pads in the 1970s – even some of the modern ones today – could not contain my flow. During the first three to four days of my period, I usually ended up either staying indoors or as close to a toilet as possible, at all times.

I was officially diagnosed with severe stage IV endometriosis at fifteen years old. The pain had become so unbearable that my mother had to make an appointment with a gynaecologist. That appointment at the gynaecologist's office still lives in my memory, as if it were just yesterday. The unpleasant procedure of a stranger doing an 'internal' examination and roughly feeling the inside of my body, as I lay there frozen to the spot dressed in my school uniform with the consultant and my mother looking down at me – it was so humiliating. Although I received an official diagnosis of endometriosis that day, I was given no explanation of why, what, or how it had taken up residence in my body. The gynaecologist merely said it was hereditary, that I was unlucky, and told me that pregnancy would cure it, or that I needed to go on the birth control pill.

Well, the gynaecologist was right about one thing; the condition I had was indeed hereditary. My mother had an extreme and severe case of endometriosis too, which began when she was young. She told me stories about how the doctors would gather around her bed in the hospital after yet another operation, excitedly expectant to observe her recovery because of the extent to which she had the disease – it had become widespread in her abdomen.

The doctors back then held firm to their belief and their theory that the condition was purely genetic. However, my grandmother never suffered from it, nor her three sisters, or any other distant female relatives. The doctors also told my mother her condition was so severe that it was unlikely she would ever have children. This would not be the first time she proved the medical professionals wrong, because she went on to give birth to my brother and me.

There is a popular train of thought within the gynaecological profession that pregnancy cures endometriosis. This theory proved incorrect for my mother, as even after having my brother and me, she was constantly going in and out of the hospital with chocolate cysts the size of oranges, and countless other cysts. In her 40s, she was 'sold' by the gynaecologist on the idea that a hysterectomy would cure her ailments for good. "No more bleeding and no more pain," he said.

They were right about the bleeding, but not about the pain. The hysterectomy operation did take away some of the old symptoms but created many new, worse ones. Despite the removal of my mother's womb, she still experienced a lot of pelvic pain due to inflammation of some of her internal organs, and no one explained this to her. It was only later that we found out that some of the endometrial tissues had already migrated outside of the womb, long before the hysterectomy. Of course, the hysterectomy did not work, and her endometriosis grew back with even greater ferocity, reigniting her old problems whilst creating new ones too.

These endometriosis tissues have an abnormal ability to grow somewhere else; hence they call endometriosis the 'Wandering Womb'. Medicine has yet to discover the real reason why. After that operation, my mother's views of doctors and consultants changed, and she would often say "doctors bury their mistakes" and "do not trust doctors". Her words would repeatedly play in my head in the coming years. They taught me to question everything the doctors told me, and instead do my own research.

Even though doctors and consultants told me many times that I would never have any children, I ultimately proved all of them wrong, as my mother had done. I first had a beautiful baby girl called Maxine, and then nine years later, despite two damaged fallopian tubes and only part of one ovary left, I gave birth to a handsome baby boy called Sebastian.

As you can see, it is so easy to look to doctors as all-knowing and knowledgeable regarding you and your body. I do believe that every doctor has the best intentions and an innate desire to help people who are suffering from ill health, but only you know your own body. You know it better than anyone else knows, and never forget that.

There are numerous reasons – such as toxins, stress, work, relationship issues, and poor health – that can affect your ability to listen to your body, which we will discuss in later chapters.

Chapter 2 -

Endometriosis Pain

* * *

Destiny is not a matter of chance; it is a matter of choice. It is not something to be waited for; but rather something to be achieved.

– William Jennings Bryan

E ndometriosis is a disease which is so profound that it can

negatively impact every single aspect of a woman's life, from the ability to control reproductive choices, to the intimate engagement in an enjoyable sex life, to the ability to plan or go about an everyday task.

Endometriosis is a painful disorder among women in which endometrium-like tissue (endometrium is the tissue that lines the inside of the uterus) grows outside of the uterus. This abnormal growth is called an endometrial implant. Endometrial implants vary widely in size, shape, and colour. Over the years, they may diminish in size or disappear, or they may grow. Early implants are usually tiny and look like clear pimples. If they continue to grow, they may form flat injured areas (called lesions), small nodules or cysts filled with a fluid called 'endometriomas', which can range from sizes smaller than a pinhead to larger than a grapefruit. This disease commonly involves areas such as the ovaries, the fallopian tubes, the bowel, and the tissue lining the pelvis. Although it is highly uncommon for endometrial tissue to spread beyond the pelvic region, it has been found in other areas of the body, as well as in animals and men.

During a normal menstrual period, the endometrial tissue which lines the inside of the uterus thickens, breaks down and bleeds, sheds, and exits the body. Some inflammatory hormones, which are known as prostaglandins, can cause cramping and discomfort, and this is medically known as dysmenorrhea. High levels of estrogen lead to the production of an excess of prostaglandin, which is a chemical messenger that causes the uterine muscles to contract. The more prostaglandin is produced, the more pain a woman will experience.

However, during a menstrual period for a woman with endometriosis, the endometrial tissue that has grown outside of the uterus and is now sat in the abdomen, continues to act as it normally should – it thickens, breaks down, sheds and bleeds – but the displaced tissue has no way to exit the body and becomes trapped.

Endometriosis in the abdomen results in internal bleeding and inflammation, which causes pain and cysts to form. The other surrounding tissue can become irritated, which may eventually cause adhesions to develop in the affected area, binding other organs together unnecessarily. Endometriosis often causes severe pelvic pain during the menstrual period – it is the primary symptom and many women I know usually experience cramping. As in my case with endometriosis, I described it as a continual appendicitis-like pain; the type that takes your breath away, makes you cry out or double up. I have also observed that endometriosis pain tends to increase and spread over time.

History

So now you know a bit more about the nature of the condition, what is its history? In ancient Greece, physicians referred to the displacement of endometrial tissue outside of the uterus as 'a wandering uterus'. The social belief was that the womb was the origin of all diseases of women, and as such it should be confined and controlled. The word 'hysteria' is derived from the Greek language, and it means womb.

Aristotle (385-322 BC) believed that hysteria was caused by a discontented uterus and excessive emotions in women, which is why he thought women were unfit to be in politics. Women had no independent existence in ancient Greece and were always under the control of their father or husband. Because of their inferior social standing, women's biology was referred to as 'bad', and therefore, their physiology was not factored into the teachings of philosophers like Aristotle. This may explain society's aversion to discussing 'women's problems' even today.

The ancient Greeks thought the womb 'moved' in situations of insufficient food, exhaustion, and menstrual suppression. Most of the physical and emotional female illnesses during that Classical Period were described as hysteria. The theory of hysteria and the myth of the wandering womb still hold force, some 2500 years later, and continue to influence medical practice and doctors today. For example, in ancient Greece, it was believed that sex and pregnancy were ultimate cures – something still promoted by today's doctors – and that when women did not have intercourse, her womb became liable to be displaced and dry.

Modern-Day Medicine

In modern-day medicine, many general practitioners (GPs) in the UK are given approximately only ten days of training in gynaecology as part of their medical training. Women with endometriosis may have put up with severe and prolonged pain over many years before they eventually go to visit their doctor. As such, the doctor may be unaware of the debilitating nature of endometriosis and may dismiss the pain and the woman as hysterical or neurotic. Naturally, this compounds the problem for women. Sometimes a doctor may perform a physical and pelvic exam after collecting a symptom report and medical history. The pelvic examination will evaluate the size and position of the ovaries and check for tender masses or nodules behind the cervix.

If the doctor believes the woman's pain, then she may be offered the birth control pill or intrauterine coil (IUD). Neither of these contraceptive methods gets to the root cause and can often create more endometriosis symptoms and side effects. The woman may be referred to have imaging tests carried out. A non-invasive ultrasound is an imaging technique which is performed in cases where other conditions are suspected as well, such as uterine fibroids, ovarian cysts, or ectopic pregnancy. Ultrasound will miss small cysts or endometrial implants but can pick up cysts larger than 1cm (about 1/3 inch). Other imaging techniques, such as computed tomography (CT) scanning or magnetic resonance imaging (MRI), may occasionally be used. The issue associated with the imaging of endometriosis is that specific training is required to identify signs – often less experienced examiners will miss these and therefore will incorrectly judge that the patient does not have endometriosis. Also, in places where medical care is not publicly funded, the cost of the procedure may be too much for women to afford.

If the woman is persistent with the doctor, then she may be referred to a gynaecologist. The gynaecologist may prescribe more potent hormonal drugs or suggest surgery. Both can have severe and life-changing side effects which are rarely explained to women.

Many women with endometriosis are left feeling so understandably desperate to get out of chronic pain that they trustingly pass over their bodies and control to people who are essentially strangers, in the hope of getting 'cured'. Medical professionals rarely explain that the treatment is merely trying to help manage symptoms, rather than address the underlying causes. This leaves the woman in an endless cycle of drugs, surgery, complications, side effects and more pain. It is clear that no woman could ever make up the intensity of pain that is endometriosis.

What is cruel, however, is that some people in the medical profession do not believe the intensity of pain described by sufferers, meaning many women with endometriosis have to 'fight' to be believed.

Chapter 3 -

Endometriosis Symptoms and Causes

* * *

Know Thyself

— *Socrates*

T he symptoms of endometriosis are many and range in

frequency and severity based on several factors. Some women with endometriosis have a belief that they can only get a diagnosis of endometriosis from a gynaecologist. Unfortunately, to get a diagnosis from a gynaecologist invariably means the woman has to have an operation, which is very damaging to her already 'pained' body. Some women go through the trauma of an operation only to have the gynaecologist say they could find nothing, leaving the woman distraught and confused. However, there are other ways to have endometriosis confirmed, and this can be by going through a list of common symptoms and a process of elimination. Make sure you find a doctor who is understanding of the condition, and who is supportive. That is particularly important. You need to have someone who believes you and who wants to work with you to approach endometriosis naturally, or at least from a different perspective than merely relying on drugs and surgery.

Change your doctor or medical practice if need be to find someone who will support you. Ideally, the doctor will initially want to discount any other issues or illnesses, and will then support your desire to approach endometriosis naturally. I will be encouraging you to listen to your body and your instincts throughout this book, and to develop confidence in your own knowledge of your body. This is important if you feel you have not been taken seriously by the medical machine before. After all, you know your body best.

Here is a list of the types of symptoms and signs that may point out whether you have, or are on the verge of having, endometriosis. It must be noted, however, that this is by no means an exhaustive list.

- Severe pelvic, lower abdominal pain that seems to get worse every menstruation. The pain may begin a day or two before, and will extend several days into the menstrual period, and may include significant lower back, vaginal, leg, and abdominal pain.

- Heavy prolonged period bleeding with clots – heavy blood flows with thick clots that may extend to 7-10 days.

- Ovulation pain – pain may be noticeable at ovulation, around day 12-14 of your cycle, when an egg is released from the ovary.

- Bowel or urinary disorders – you may experience painful bowel movements or urination, or bladder pressure within your menstrual period. Irritable bowel syndrome, constipation, or diarrhoea is common.

- Painful sexual intercourse – pain during or after having sex is a common symptom with endometriosis. You may be unable to climax or have spotting or bleeding after sex.

- Infertility – often, women who seek infertility treatment are diagnosed with endometriosis.

- Other symptoms may also be signs of having endometriosis: spotting during your cycle, abnormal pap smear, chronic debilitating fatigue/chronic fatigue syndrome (CFS), fibromyalgia, premenstrual tension (PMT), allergies, migraines, restless leg syndrome, insomnia, night sweats, hot flushes, breast tenderness, water retention, bloating or nausea that tends to worsen every menstrual period.

Diagnosis

Suppose you have two or more of the above symptoms, and have ruled out any other possible causes with your doctor (i.e., blood tests for other conditions have come back clear), then, in that case, it is highly probable that endometriosis is the cause.

Medical professionals or GPs will invariably try to prescribe hormonal drugs, or refer you to a gynaecological consultant to have the diagnosis of endometriosis validated by surgical means. Also, do be aware that many doctors will dismiss your symptoms, or potentially wrongly diagnose you with another condition. Similarly, gynaecologists may not give a diagnosis if they do not find any endometriosis even if there are signs that you are suffering from the condition. In fact, this tends to be more common than getting a diagnosis – on average it takes about seven and a half years from the onset of symptoms for women to get a diagnosis.[3] That is a considerable amount of time to be suffering with no name for your predicament.

However, even if you do get a diagnosis do not underestimate how both types of proposed treatments – drugs and surgery – can carry great long-term, irreversible risks and side effects that can permanently damage the body. Pharmaceuticals merely try and manage the symptoms of endometriosis but do not address the underlying causes of the condition. Painkillers, drugs, and surgery may mask symptoms rather than address the underlying root causes. Therefore the process of elimination from the above checklist and a consultation with your doctor may be all you need to believe you have the condition.

Although severe pelvic pain is the primary symptom of endometriosis, it is not always a reliable indicator of the extent of the endometriosis condition. I have met some women with only mild endometriosis but who experience extensive pain, while I have met others with advanced endometriosis who experience only a little discomfort. Therefore, it is essential to carefully observe and pay keen attention to everything you experience during every one of your menstrual periods. It would be useful to record your pain scores and symptoms in a journal or on a mobile app. You will want this information to monitor your progress as you move through the book and start adapting the changes I suggest.

Causes

The definitive causes of endometriosis remain in debate and are still not certain. As such it is frequently referred to as the 'disease of theories'. No single researcher or medical practitioner has found the exact answer, but several theories have been put forward. I will explain each of them below:

- Retrograde menstruation – this is one of the most highly favoured explanations for endometriosis. Here, it is proposed that during retrograde menstruation, the menstrual blood, which contains endometrial cells, flows back up through the fallopian tubes and into the pelvic cavity instead of out of the body. These displaced cells will then stick to the pelvic walls and surfaces of the other pelvic organs, where they will grow and continue to thicken and bleed throughout each menstrual period. Although most medical practitioners generally accept this as the main culprit for endometriosis, there is still no explanation as to why the displaced tissue flows backwards.

- Immune system or immunologic dysfunction – it is also possible that a 'broken' immune system or any problems with it can make the body unable to recognise and eliminate the endometrial tissue that is growing outside the uterus.

- Embryonic cell growth – all of the cells lining the pelvic and abdominal cavities come from embryonic cells. Whenever one or more of the small areas of the abdominal lining turn into endometrial tissue, endometriosis can and may develop.

- Transport of endometrial cells – another rare possibility, where the lymphatic system of blood vessels and tissue fluids may transport the endometrial cells to other parts of the body.

- Genetics – another favoured theory states there is a 70% risk of women and girls inheriting the disease if their mothers or female relatives have endometriosis.

- Environmental factors – toxins referred to as xenoestrogens and phytoestrogens have been known to cause cell changes and mutations, which cause immune disorders and allow for implantation of menstrual debris. Some 51 xenoestrogen chemicals have been found to disrupt human hormonal balance. Tampons, for example, contain traces of dioxins, although they may state they are made of 100% natural cotton. Xenoestrogens are found in many aspects of our everyday life via pesticide sprayed food, household products and personal care products. Phytoestrogens are the most studied of all the phytochemicals and are weaker than the natural estrogen hormones. Although not as potent as other forms of estrogen mimickers, it is best to avoid them. They are found in things like soy and wheat.

- Dioxins – dioxins are a by-product of chlorinated products and plastics, and second in line to radioactive waste. A draft report released in September 1994 by the US Environmental Protection Agency describes dioxin as a serious public health threat. There is a wealth of research showing the effects of toxins like dioxins on women and how they can lead to endometriosis. In 1993, rhesus monkeys were exposed, over ten years, to low levels of TCDD (2,3,7,8-Tetrachlorodibenzo-p-dioxin), which is a colourless compound without a distinguishable odour. These monkeys subsequently developed reproductive abnormalities and endometriosis.[4] TCDD is known to be a human carcinogen, and human exposure is greater than the levels that the monkeys were exposed to in the experiment. Many studies have found women with endometriosis have significant levels of dioxins indicated in their bodies.

- Implantation through surgical scar – Although this is a rare occurrence, it is possible. What typically happens is after a surgery such as a hysterectomy or a cesarean section, endometrial cells may attach to the surgical incision.

These theories have become a foundation for diagnosing women with endometriosis. Nevertheless, there are still other factors that would increase the risk of getting the disease. One such factor, that is favoured by the medical profession, is never giving birth. This theory is based mainly on the premise that almost none of the women who had children before the 1970s had endometriosis. However, I believe the leading cause behind this to be the greater prevalence of various forms of toxicity in our environment (what I refer to as the five poisons or five Ps – produce, products, property, people, and past). I will cover this in more detail later.

There are other factors that have yet to be mentioned: a long history of pelvic infections, abnormalities in the uterus, severe prolonged stress and any medical condition that prevents the normal passage of menstrual flow out of the body. Endometriosis is known to develop a few years after the onset of menstruation but this is not always true – it was not the case with me. The signs and symptoms of this disease may cease temporarily with pregnancy and sometimes end with menopause, but not always.

Endometriosis can cause many complications including those listed below:

Infertility

The main complication that endometriosis brings is infertility, or a difficulty in getting pregnant or not being able to get pregnant at all. About 30% to 50% of women with endometriosis have difficulty getting pregnant.[5] One reason for this is that endometriosis can damage the fallopian tubes or the ovaries, which will cause fertility problems.

For pregnancy to occur, first, an egg is released from an ovary, and it will travel down through the neighbouring fallopian tube. Next, a sperm cell will come along to attempt to fertilise the egg cell. Once it is successful, the fertilised egg will attach itself to the wall of the uterus to begin development. An endometriosis condition may obstruct the passage in the fallopian tube and keep the egg and sperm from uniting.

In some cases, the condition also seems to affect fertility in less direct ways, such as to cause damage to the sperm or egg cell.

Despite this, it is estimated that up to 70% of women who have mild to moderate conditions of endometriosis can still conceive and will be able to get pregnant without the help of treatment.[6] Treatment using medication does not guarantee the improvement of fertility in women with endometriosis. Surgery to remove the visible patches of the endometriosis implants is sometimes considered, but then again this too does not give a guarantee that you will get pregnant and in fact, often the pelvic region develops yet more adhesions. Due to the difficulty of dealing with this disease, doctors often advise women with endometriosis not to delay having children as the condition usually worsens with time.

Ovarian Cysts

The other main complication brought about by endometriosis is ovarian cysts. These start as small fluid-filled cysts on the ovaries that are brought about when the endometriosis tissue grows near the ovaries. They may be colourless, red, or very dark brown. When these ovarian cysts, otherwise known as endometriomas or 'chocolate cysts', are filled with thick, old, dark brown blood, they can grow large and become incredibly painful. If the cyst bursts then the contents can spill out or empty all over the abdominal cavity and organs, causing excruciating pain.

Adhesions

The inflammatory condition and nature of endometriosis can cause repeated scar tissue to form, called adhesions. Adhesions are of a similar appearance to the thin white chicken skin. They cause an organ to stick or be pulled together with another organ, causing intense pain.

For example, they may cause the intestines (bowel) or bladder to attach to the abdominal wall. These dense, web-like structures of scar tissue can cause significant pelvic pain, impairing the quality of life, work, and social activities.

There is a common misconception that cysts and adhesions complications can be removed by surgery. However, the surgery causes more trauma to the pelvis, and more adhesions. In a high percentage of women, their endometriosis symptoms often reoccur in a matter of weeks following the surgery. This can be very disheartening for a woman with endometriosis to have undergone the trauma of an operation, only to discover that it has been unsuccessful. The woman is back to square one with very few options and stuck in the maze of the medical machine.

Chapter 4 -

The Medical Machine

* * *

*The greatest pleasure in life is doing what people say you cannot
do*

— Walter Bagehot

The medical establishments in the Western world have

developed some incredible ways to combat illness and diseases, which
has in turn improved our quality of life and enabled us to live for
longer. The intent to combat illness has led to the growth and increased
use of pharmaceutical drugs, which in many aspects has been highly
successful. We have made some great quantum leaps in our health care
and generally we reap the rewards. For example, the transplanting of
hearts, livers, and kidneys (to name a few body parts) and the incredible
life-saving endeavours of the accident and emergency departments in
hospitals. No longer is there any worry of dying in childbirth or
succumbing to diseases like smallpox or measles. The discovery and
development of antibiotics, in particular, has been beneficial for many,
although increasingly governments and medical organisations are
becoming aware that their effectiveness is declining from overuse. The

general population has come to expect antibiotics for almost everything – even the common cold (against which antibiotics are entirely ineffective as it is a viral, not bacterial, infection). Due to the abundance of toxins and poisons in our environment, many individuals have weaker immune systems, meaning they must take antibiotics repeatedly or over extended periods. Overuse of antibiotics and drugs has led to the development of immunities, chemical sensitivities, and allergies. Critically, it has also had an untold detrimental effect on many people's organs, body systems and their own natural defence system – the immune system.

The human body is an amazing machine in itself. Our intestines (bowel), for example, has its own 'good' gut bacteria that combats any pathogens that may enter the body through the mouth and move into the digestive tract. Excess use of drugs and antibiotics kill off this gut bacteria, thereby leaving the body vulnerable to yet more infections. Whilst modern medicine has achieved many incredible feats, the Western world has become increasingly unwell, and the prescription of chemical treatments has become commonplace. Pharmaceutical giants carry significant influence over medical establishments and governments, and one has to question the overuse of chemical treatments, and what natural remedies were used before their invention.

One must also appreciate that whilst certain types of diseases have receded under the dominion of modern medicine, other types of illness like cancers, and cardiovascular and autoimmune diseases have grown considerably. Now, not all of this can be attributed to modern medicine but we have to wonder why we are, as a population, still getting more and more ill despite the 'advances' in medicine and the billions of dollars invested every year. What we can take from this is two-fold – that modern medicine is not working for many diseases (if anything it is making some diseases worse), and that our current environment is getting too toxic. As mentioned earlier, one big issue with much of modern medicine is that the drugs and surgery they prescribe only address symptoms and not the root causes.

Let us take coronary heart disease, for example. The treatment for this disease is drugs like statins and surgery. However, for the majority of sufferers, heart disease is not caused by a deficiency in statins – it is down to their lifestyle and environment. As such a prudent approach would be for sufferers to improve their diet, exercise more and try to reduce stress. Of course, this may not work for everyone as some cases of heart disease are caused by other factors and not just your environment, but in general it would be far more effective than drugs or surgery. What many people do not realise is your body does not just get ill – for the most part, there is something external causing it. There is a reason behind every illness and a reason why your body is not able to fight it.

For some diseases like cancer, some radical approaches are taken from chemotherapy to removal of the affected area or organ. However, conditions like endometriosis are harder to diagnose as women may have an array of symptoms. An inexperienced doctor may carry out blood tests, find no 'abnormal' results and conclude that the women with endometriosis are either 'making it up' or neurotic. The woman may be dismissed as imagining or exaggerating the pain and prescribed some or any of the following array of pharmaceuticals: pain killers, nonsteroidal anti-inflammatory drugs (NSAIDs), oral contraceptives, an intrauterine device (IUD) like Mirena coil, NuvaRing, deposhot, or some other synthetic hormone to manipulate the ability to conceive. However, these hormone manipulators prevent ovulation from occurring, so fewer hormones, like progesterone, are produced – thus continuing the body's hormonal imbalance.

Listed below are some of the current medical treatment options that a woman with endometriosis may be routinely offered when she visits her doctor, physician or gynaecologist. This list is a guide and not exclusive:

- Tens machine

- Birth control pill/oral contraceptives

- Mirena coil/IUD

- Antidepressants

- Painkillers/nonsteroidal anti-inflammatory drugs (NSAIDs); paracetamol, ibuprofen, dihydrocodeine, codeine

- Postap

- Danazol

- Zoladex

- Oramorph

- Propolis

- Cerezette

- Decapeptyl injections

- Pain blockers

- Womb biopsy

- Morphine patches

- Shrinking cyst on ovary

- Cystectomy

- Abdominal ablation

- Excision surgery

- Diagnostic laparoscopy

- Hysterectomy – full removal of uterus and ovaries which results in instant menopause and in the long term possible osteoporosis

- Opherectomy – removal of uterus leaving ovaries, resulting in a slow menopause and subsequent surgery when ovaries die off due to insufficient blood supply

- Hormonal Treatments – there are over 40 different types of birth control pills which consist of a variety of synthetic estrogen compounds and synthetic progesterone called 'progestin'.

It is important to note, and repeat, that none of the drugs or hormonal treatments prescribed will eliminate endometriosis. Current medical treatment aims to reduce inflammation and tries to manage symptoms. However, this rarely happens, and a lot of women may end up having severe side effects and complications. The idea of hormone treatment, with the use of synthetic hormones, is to trick the pituitary gland into believing you have reached menopause.

- Synthetic progestogen and progestins. This is important but can be confusing to a lot of women; these products 'progestogen' and 'progestins' are NOT natural bioidentical progesterone. (*Note how similar the chemical synthetic pharmaceutical names are to progesterone which you produce in your body.) Some synthetic progestogen hormone drugs prescribed are called norethisterone, dydrogesterone and medroxyprogesterone.

- GnRH analogues – these are synthetic gonadotrophin-releasing hormones that mimic the three gonadotropins that the body produces: luteinizing hormone, follicle-stimulating hormone and chorionic gonadotropin. Some drugs are;

Buserelin, Nafarelin, Goserelin and Lupron. All these drugs cause serious side effects and in particular Lupron which has been known to cause severe long term damage to the body.

- Mirena Coil/IUD/levonorgestrel intrauterine system is a small 'T' shaped device inserted into the uterus to provide a slow release of synthetic progestin over several years. Side effects are ovarian cysts, pelvic pain, weight gain, irregular bleeding, spotting, mood swings, thin and brittle hair. Pelvic infections are common due to the 'string' that hangs down from the coil. The uterus is usually kept sterile, but the string increases the likelihood of infection. Other side effects are extreme pain and bleeding during intercourse if the coil is dislodged.

Almost all of the listed treatments can cause an array of side effects, with some being very severe and life-changing. By way of example, let us look at the side effects of birth control pills and hormonal drugs:

- Growth of hair on chin, upper lip, breasts, inner thighs and abdomen
- Excessive weight gain
- Acne
- Deepening of voice
- Depression
- Cardiovascular problems
- Heart attacks
- Damage to the digestive system
- Leg swellings
- Damage to the reproductive system

- Hair thinning and hair loss

- Vomiting

- Nausea

- Bloating

- Spotting

- Headaches and migraines

- Mood swings

- Breast tenderness

- Water retention

- Blood clots

- Dizziness

This is by no means an exhaustive list either. There are many other side effects not listed here that women on these drug treatments may experience.

Some of these side effects are irreversible, and in some cases, side effects are treated with yet more drugs – which cause more side effects. And so the cycle continues.

I visited numerous doctors and gynaecologists over the years and was offered many of the above painkillers, drugs, and surgical options. However, no one ever discussed any other alternatives with me – they just promoted one drug or hormonal treatment after the next. By the time I had my second child, the medical profession had referred to my uterus as if it were a redundant organ that needed removing. It was talked about as if there was no other use for it because I was over the age of 40. One gynaecologist even said, "*I am not sure it is necessary for you to keep it.*" It was as though he was referring to an empty crisp packet that might be thrown in the waste paper basket. I was outraged that an essential female sex organ could be regarded so dismissively. Whilst the uterus' primary purpose is for childbearing, it also serves the critical function of providing structural integrity and support for the bladder, bowel, pelvic bones, and organs. Primarily this involves separating the bowel and bladder. If the uterus is removed, it can cause the surrounding organs to collapse away from their regular positions, thus leading to injury and pain. There are a whole host of other side effects too such as early menopause, blood clots, infections, pain during sexual intercourse, anaesthesia problems (breathing or heart problems), and heavy bleeding to name just a few. The doctors knew about all these likely outcomes but yet were still so eagerly willing to remove my uterus.

What bothered me the most was that women could be put under pressure to make important decisions about drugs and the life-changing surgical removal of a vital organ when they are in great distress and pain. The woman may also be in a vulnerable position. She might be lying in pain in the hospital bed, full of drugs and painkillers, with no makeup on and wearing a thin cotton gown, unable to think clearly. This is not the ideal situation to be making life-changing decisions or not be fully informed of the risks. Your uterus is a sacred organ, and it is essential for a woman's health that it be retained.

There are many current treatments for endometriosis through the medical machine. Still, the real, undisclosed fact is NONE of these common drugs and treatments addresses the root causes or underlying triggers of endometriosis. What I did find interesting through my research was that fifty years ago, the pharmaceutical giants were not so prominent. The principles were quite different from today and doctors in the 1960s, in the USA and UK, would routinely prescribe natural treatments like bioidentical progesterone cream. This was a particularly effective treatment at reducing symptoms and had no side effects. So why did no doctor offer natural bioidentical progesterone cream to me as an option?

You may find that some doctors you interact with are stubborn, condescending, or hostile. You may find it challenging to speak up, suggest other alternatives or ask for a new doctor. But you must stand up for yourself and your body. Below is a little list to help you find your voice and deal with any bullying doctors.

Do's and Don'ts with Doctors and Physicians

Be confident and don't be scared to ask lots of questions when visiting your doctor or physician. Do consider making written notes, or ask to record the meeting on your mobile phone when discussing any aspect relating to drugs or surgery. When you are in incredible pain, taking strong pain killers or unable to sleep, you may have a fuzzy head and find it difficult to remember or take in any new information you are being given.

Take a trusted friend or family member with you. Many times I took a friend or family member with me, and it made a big difference to how I was treated and how confident I felt in asking questions. In fact, on visiting a gynaecologist for a second time, I took my partner. The gynaecologist then went on to prescribe and promote a different drug to what he had suggested in my first meeting with him (although I later decided to take neither). The list of side effects to the drugs he was recommending was far too disturbing and disruptive to my already pained body.

When you are fully informed about your body, and anything you are going to have put in it, or any trauma carried out to it, you are at an enormous advantage and far more likely to make the right decisions and be under no illusions. Ideally, you will reject the conventional medical route and decide the safer option is to move forward towards approaching endometriosis using a more natural approach. The natural approach helps identify the sources of pain and to eliminate them. I hope you have realised that painkillers, drugs and surgery only try to manage the symptoms of endometriosis and neglect to address the underlying causes.

If only I had been informed of this many, many years ago.

Chapter 5 -

Is Approaching Endometriosis 'Naturally' Really an Option?

* * *

Two roads diverged in a wood, and I.....I took the one less travelled by, and that has made all the difference

– Robert Frost

Endometriosis had caused me issues since my first

menstruation, but after the birth of my son, it got progressively worse. I made regular visits to the gynaecologist, who suggested that I take various oral contraceptives, coils and pharmaceutical drugs. The gynaecologist reassured me they would stop my menstrual cycle and 'may' help me with the pain. However, I had been pregnant for nine months without a menstrual cycle, and my symptoms had worsened. So what had gone wrong? I researched online about the side effects to the prescription drugs he was proposing, and they were disturbing, and in some cases irreversible. I decided to see if there was an alternative route. I just kept thinking, "there has to be another way!"

It was Hippocrates (460-370 BC) – often referred to as the 'father of medicine' – who sought out natural explanations for natural phenomena, and who taught that natural means could be employed to fight disease. Although I do not necessarily recommend this, Hippocrates suggested the rubbing of honey on the vagina and the chewing of cloves of garlic as ancient treatments prescribed to 'lure the uterus back to its seat'. This all seemed peculiar to me, but I decided to do some more investigating.

My research led me to this statement: "If you cut out wheat from your diet your symptoms will disappear." (Referred to as The Endometriosis Diet).

I could not quite believe what I was reading. Was it that simple? Could the removal of wheat remove the pain? I sat there at the computer with a prescription in my hand. The internet was full of stories and warned there could be many possible side effects to the drug I had been prescribed. I had two options now; cut out wheat or take these prescribed drugs. I was aware something had to change. I could not carry on with the level of pain I was experiencing. However, I was not prepared to swap one set of symptoms with other, more disturbing, irreversible ones. Something had to give. Could something so simple as removing wheat from my diet work? I thought, "What the heck, it is worth a try! What is the worst thing that can happen? At least I know excluding a food product has no side effects."

After doing further research, I found out that wheat was genetically modified in the early 1970s in order for the head of the wheat to contain more kernels. However, this made the plant top-heavy, and thus caused the crop to fall over. So, to solve this issue, a hormone was injected into wheat to thicken the stalk. Again, a problem occurred – the thicker stalks meant the wheat grew closer together, which allowed a fungus to spread between the stems. This led to another hormone being added to destroy the fungus. It is possible that these two hormones (as well as toxic pesticides like Roundup that are sprayed on wheat), when absorbed in excess, upset the hormone profiles of women with endometriosis.[7]

I focused on what was essential for me, and that was getting out of pain. It was suggested that the removal of wheat from my diet might attain that. However, to remove wheat from my diet involved quite a significant mental shift for me.

My idea of a healthy diet before was, in fact, completely unhealthy. I lived out of local bakeries. I ate fruit scones for breakfast, grazed on sugar items throughout the day, and my idea of a vegetable was iceberg lettuce (which is mainly composed of water and has a weak nutritional profile). Instead, I should have been eating leafy greens, cruciferous vegetables and even the more nutritious types of lettuce like romaine and red leaf. I knew nothing of healthy eating. But my motivation was to get well, educate myself and take full responsibility for my own body. I did not want to take body-altering drugs with horrible side effects. The definition of insanity is doing the same thing over and over and expecting different results; I had to do something differently.

When I went wheat-free in the year 2001, there were no commercially available wheat- or gluten-free products on the market. Even though I was a novice in the kitchen, I learnt how to make all sorts of loaves of bread, like sweet potato bread, and stocked up the cupboards with packets of oatcakes and rice cakes. I always carried emergency packets of oatcakes in my handbag in case I was stuck somewhere with no food options that I could eat. I used to find the prospect of going out to eat so complicated, and then people would look at me as if I were an alien when I said I was wheat intolerant. I dropped the 'intolerance' name and soon changed it to 'allergy', which in time stopped the strange questioning looks.

I had the odd quivering bottom lip when I would turn up to a cafe or restaurant to find all the main meals had wheat flour in it, and there was nothing but potatoes, rice, or fruit for me to eat. Although nowadays it is easier and far more enjoyable to eat out as restaurants and cafes are increasingly more aware and accommodating to our wheat-free (and now gluten-free, dairy-free, nut-free etc.) dietary needs. There are even sections of supermarket aisles fully dedicated to carrying wheat-free and gluten-free products, which I still find exciting to this day!

Therefore, the commitment was made and, although it was hard to adjust my eating habits and diet initially, within a few months, I felt a significant reduction in pain at ovulation and menstruation. My periods became a 2-3 day affair, rather than 7-10 days as they had been previously, and the blood flow became minimal with absolutely no clots. I was ecstatic! Slowly but surely, as the weeks turned into months and I began to accommodate my new eating regime, I was able to confidently start planning and living a normal life again.

I returned to the gynaecologist and shared with him the exciting developments, encouraging him to share my experience and success with other women. His response, however, was that he could not share it with his other patients, as 'it was not proven through the National Institute of Clinical Excellence (NICE) guidelines'. The message was loud and clear; the medical establishment would be happy to put me on drugs with life-changing, and damaging side effects that would keep me in a hamster wheel of symptoms, but would not even consider a dietary change suggestion. I was aghast.

I learnt later about all the money and influence the pharmaceutical companies have. Pharmaceuticals is a massive industry, with the total industry value estimated at $1.2 trillion and set to exceed $1.5 trillion by 2023.[8] Yes, worth repeating: over $1.2 trillion a year in sales. Pharmaceuticals and drugs are BIG business. But what about all the poor, trusting women who are not told about the real impact of the side effects of these drugs, or about how they do not 'cure' or put endometriosis into remission?

These drugs keep them trapped in a vicious 'medical machine', in a maze of chemicals that end up causing them lifelong damage and do nothing to address the underlying causes. The majority of drugs now are just used to make money; to bolster the already enormous revenue of pharmaceutical companies. Very few drugs have a net positive impact on the patients they are supposedly meant to help – yes they might mask some symptoms but is that worth developing other conditions and side effects? Even if we are told that some drugs are safe and effective in many instances, this is not the case. Medical science is tethered to the pharmaceutical industry's hunt for greater profits. Often they have pumped millions of dollars and a lot of time into the development of a drug, so they have a lot to lose. Many books and scientists have attested to the fact that pharmaceuticals cherry-pick data and manipulate results to get their drugs on the market.

My gynaecologist later admitted that he had just spent ten days in an all-expenses-paid seminar in Rome, Italy. It was paid for by the pharmaceutical company who developed the drug he had been promoting to me. I also learnt that doctors got £100 per intrauterine device (IUD) inserted into a woman. It felt dirty, sordid, and wrong. I wondered at what point did the focus of medicine switch from improving people's health to making money?

Chapter 6 -

You Are What You Eat....

* * *

When the going gets tough, the tough get going
— Joseph P Kennedy

Removing wheat from my diet, and swapping it out for

healthier, fresh alternatives, was for me the first significant step to pain reduction. Within a few months, my pain score had reduced by almost 50%. The difference in my body surprised me as it was so simple, yet it was a profoundly effective course of action.

However, on one occasion I ate a small amount of wheat, and within ten minutes, the pain hit my abdomen hard. It was now apparent to me that excluding wheat not only helped with the elimination of my menstrual cycle pain and a reduction in bleeding but also with the old bloating and distention of my stomach. Ovulation and menstruation started to come and go without incident. I began to feel like I could make social plans again, spend time with my children, put the hot water bottle away in the cupboard and stop feeling like a bystander in my life. What a massive difference to the quality of my

life wheat removal made. This one small change made a BIG
ˌdifference.

Why Wheat?

Ever since grain spread to Europe in 5000-3700 BC, bread has always
been a large part of our Western diet. Even nowadays, especially during
breakfast, lunch or dinner, our meal seems incomplete without bread.
In fact, it is not only bread we need to watch out for; we should be
careful not to eat too much of anything that contains ingredients from
grains. Why is this so? Grains, specifically gluten-containing and
refined ones (but in some cases also unrefined, gluten-free grains), can
cause irritation and inflammation in your gut.[9]

Nowadays, many factors have meant that there is far more
gluten in wheat too. Bread contains more gluten nowadays due to
modern baking practices which involve smaller fermentation periods.[10]
Also, the mechanisation of farming and increased use of pesticides,
nitrogen fertiliser and agrochemicals has led to the development of
more toxic gluten peptides.[11]

There are a lot of other grains, but why focus only on wheat?
There are three main culprits here – gluten, wheat germ agglutinin
(WGA) and opioid peptides (specifically gluten exorphins found in
wheat) – all of these are harmful to your body, and all of these are
found in wheat, with two of them exclusive to this grain.

So what are they?

Gluten is a group of proteins comprised of prolamins, mainly glutelin
and gliadin. Around 80% of wheat is composed of gluten. Wheat germ
agglutinin is a lectin. Lectins serve a multitude of purposes, but they
primarily act as a defensive system and a deterrent to organisms and

predators like insects, which therefore helps to protect the grain. They also help with communication between cells. Opioid peptides is the general term for enkephalins, endorphins and dynorphins. These peptides are made naturally in the body and act as hormones and neuromodulators. They can also be found externally in foods like wheat (gluten exorphins) and are also mimicked by opiates and opioids.

Why are they so bad for me?

Gluten sensitivity has been estimated to affect up to 13% of the world's population, with a further 1.4% suffering from coeliac disease.[12] However, given the toxicity of gluten and our environment, those figures are likely to be even higher. As mentioned previously, gliadin is one of the dominant proteins in gluten. The issue here is it also causes multiple problems in the body. This is down to its peptide chains, which are highly resistant to the gastric, pancreatic and intestinal enzymes in the gastrointestinal tract.[13] The results of this are inflammation and digestive issues.

Several other proteins within gluten are also reported to be immunogenic and thus cause inflammation. Gluten's inflammatory effect in the gut can also cause intestinal cells to die prematurely, which will inevitably lead to leaky gut, thus enabling bacterial proteins and toxic compounds to get into the bloodstream. This damage to the intestinal lining can cause further digestive issues and make it harder to absorb necessary nutrients.

Wheat Germ Agglutinin (WGA) – WGA is a lectin, and therefore it can cause a whole host of issues for those who ingest wheat. In fact, WGA can do direct damage to the majority of tissues in the human body without requiring a specific set of genetic susceptibilities or immune-mediated articulations. In other words, almost all humans are vulnerable to the toxicity of lectins. The reason behind this is that the two glycoproteins that WGA specifically targets (N-Acetylglucosamine and sialic acid) happen to be very much present in almost every organism on the planet. This makes WGA nature's natural pest resistance tool. The issue for humans here is that WGA, due to its affinity for those two glycoproteins mentioned above, can disrupt and gain entry to all our mucosal surfaces – all the way from our nasal cavities, to our blood vessels. It has also been shown to be pro-inflammatory, immunotoxic, neurotoxic, cytotoxic, cardiotoxic, as well as to interfere with endocrine function, gene expression and gastrointestinal function.

What is more, humans over thousands of years have been selectively breeding wheat to increase the concentration of this protein, so nowadays our wheat is incredibly saturated with WGA, making its effects even worse. By way of example to show how prominent this issue is, in the US alone $250 million worth of glucosamine is sold annually. Glucosamine is mainly derived from the exoskeletons of organisms like shrimp, which contain large amounts of the two glycoproteins WGA binds to. The reason why so much of this supplement is sold is that it makes Americans feel better. It is not because they are deficient in the crushed up exoskeletons of crustaceans but simply because by taking it, the vast amounts of WGA Americans consume will bind to the glucosamine rather than their cells.[14]

Opioid peptides – The opioid peptides found in wheat, which are remarkably similar to opioid peptides found in opium, are known to cause addiction to wheat, and this is why withdrawal symptoms occur upon the removal of wheat from the diet. It has also been reported that these opioid peptides help to essentially anaesthetise us to the effects of WGA – hence why many people can feel okay eating wheat for some time despite the havoc it is wreaking upon the body. These opioid peptides were also noted to be a promoter of schizophrenia, and schizophrenics often see their symptoms reduce by a lot when they remove wheat from their diets.[15]

Therefore, when it comes to things that we as humans should not eat nowadays, wheat and gluten are probably at the top of the list. Although we can indulge ourselves in less healthy choices once in a while without negative consequences, wheat and all other gluten-containing grains should be avoided, especially for those of us who suffer from endometriosis and have very sensitive bodies.

I know that cutting out wheat and gluten may feel a daunting prospect. I remember feeling close to tears once when we were out at a friend's house as I did not know what to eat because everything seemed to have wheat in it – even some ice creams, sauces and sausages. This just made mealtimes so stressful for me.

I had a young family and did not want to spend hours thinking or preparing food. I was not a natural, comfortable cook. At times, I felt overwhelmed, even at the thought of eating. However, I got into juicing organic vegetables, as I found that it was an easy way to get the number of vegetables suggested. I bought some simple cookbooks and tried to adopt an approach to food that perhaps my great grandmother or my cavewoman ancestors would have had. My new philosophy was to keep it simple, fresh, free-range, organic, and to avoid processed readymade meals filled with additives.

Soups were easy to make, and when I used organic vegetables, even my children commented on how good they tasted. One of my favourite soup recipes involved a bag of frozen peas, a chopped up organic onion, a vegetable stock cube, salt, pepper, all mixed into one litre of water. Bring it all to the boil, blend and 'voila'! A yummy, tasty, inexpensive, and quick soup loved by all. There are so many other options and alternatives out there nowadays that very much allow you to still enjoy mealtimes and to eat out with friends and family.

Sugar-Free

Another aspect of my diet that needed adjustment was my sugar consumption. As I mentioned previously, I had survived my days by being pumped up on sugar, and I used to graze on the stuff all day long. Why sugar-free? Well, added sugar, the 'sweet poison' of the modern world as some experts would say, is one of the single worst ingredients in our diet. Our body does not need much sugar; in fact, sugar is a non-essential macronutrient. We can get energy from fats and complex carbohydrates. We should, as adults, only have a maximum of 30g (seven sugar cubes' worth) of added sugars daily. The fact is many people surpass this maximum recommendation by a long way; the average American consumes over three times the 30g guideline every day, whilst the average Briton consumes double the guideline amount.[16] Many do so without even realising. When we eat foods that contain added sugar or are high in sugar, we disrupt the sugar balance in our body – our blood sugar levels get disturbed. We should always avoid added sugar as if it is the plague. Below I will cover some key reasons why.

Added sugar, like sucrose and high fructose corn syrup, for example, does not contain any essential nutrients, just a whole bunch of calories. This is the reason they are called 'empty' calories. There are no proteins, essential fats, vitamins, or minerals whatsoever. Just pure energy. Sugar is also bad for your teeth because when it combines with the saliva and bacteria in your mouth, plaque is formed. Extended periods with plaque on your teeth can cause it to dissolve your enamel and thereby give you cavities.

Glucose is found in all living cells on the planet. If we cannot get it from our diet, our body produces it by converting glycogen to glucose or by harvesting amino acids and waste products. Fructose is a different case. Our body does not produce it in any significant amount, and there is no physiological need for it. This sugar originally came from fruit and makes up 55% of table sugar (sucrose). It is now used frequently as an ingredient in sweetened products (high fructose corn syrup). The issue with fructose is that it is sweeter than glucose and therefore more addictive. Also, it is harder to digest than glucose, and thus more can end up in the liver, which can lead to a cascade of metabolic issues.[17]

One of these issues is 'insulin resistance', that can lead to the development of type 2 diabetes. Insulin is a vital hormone in our body because it allows blood sugar (glucose) to travel to cells from the bloodstream by increasing their permeability to the sugar. It also promotes glycogenesis (the formation of glycogen from sugar) and lipogenesis (the metabolic formation of fat). Consuming too much sugar causes an overproduction of the insulin hormone, which can, in some cases, lead to insulin resistance. As such, cells can no longer absorb glucose and the liver will cease converting glucose into glycogen, meaning that glucose levels can reach dangerously high levels in the blood. Diabetes may also result in obesity and heart disease.

Cancer is one of the world's leading causes of death. It is characterised by uncontrolled growth and multiplication of cancerous cells. Cancer has been strongly associated with individuals who have an overproduction of insulin in their bodies. This overproduction comes from excessive consumption of sugar. For example, in one study of over 93,000 women, those who had the highest levels of insulin had more than double the risk of breast and uterine cancer years later, compared to the women with the lowest levels.[18]

Why is it so hard to resist eating sweet food? The reason for this is because sugar can cause a massive dopamine release in our brain, which, in turn, creates an addiction to it. Therefore, it takes a lot of will power to discipline ourselves and avoid eating food that contains added sugar. Notice how naturally sweet foods like fruit and milk are not nearly as addictive as sweets, chocolate, fizzy drinks, junk food etc. That is because these processed foods are filled with multiple types of sugars, and greater quantities of them. We should always instil in our minds the harmful effects of too much sugar in our body. This way, we can achieve something that truly works for healthy living – the abstinence from added sugar and reducing overall sugar intake.

Now all the negative things associated with wheat and sugar have been fully explained, I urge you to be aware of what you buy. There is a lot of conflicting nutritional advice about what to avoid and what to eat, and sometimes it can create confusion and frustration. The bottom line is to keep your awareness up and read the ingredients list at all times.

Stone Age Diet

Dr Sarah Myhill is a wonderful and inspiring doctor based in Wales, UK, whose speciality is to help people heal from chronic fatigue syndrome (CFS/ME). I learned to follow Dr Sarah Myhill's advice: "*If we simply want to stay well, we should all move towards eating a 'Stone Age' diet based on protein (meat, fish, eggs), healthy fats, nuts and fruit and vegetables. Western diets get 70% of their calories from wheat, dairy products, sugar and potato, and it is no surprise that these are the major causes of modern ill health such as cancer, heart disease, diabetes, obesity and degenerative disorders.*"

I could understand the image of a caveman in Stone Age times chasing and killing his supper and dragging it home fresh. It made sense that food was supposed to be natural, pesticide-free, additive-free or hormone-free, and importantly, not processed or packaged in plastic in a factory and travelled to more countries than me. That was what I sought for my family and me. The phrase "You are what you eat" rang through my head. If I ate rubbish, then I noticed that I felt like rubbish. When I ate healthily, I felt healthy. I could feel the difference.

So I started eating fresh and organic fruit and vegetables over the non-organic variety. Despite what some naysayers say you really can taste the difference, and it is worth the minimal difference in cost. I would sometimes juice vegetables if I found it hard to eat the recommended seven a day, or use a 'macro greens' product (wheat-free of course) which I put into a drink for an extra body boost.

Choose what works for you and remember that little changes can make a big difference, but try to avoid – where you can – chemically sprayed, bland tasting, mainstream vegetables.

I also started eating mostly free-range, organic, and grass-fed meat and poultry. The difference in taste and texture was noticeable. As my taste buds improved, I started to feel better within my body. I took full advantage of the brilliant online shopping and delivery services offered by most supermarkets. Nowadays, the options available online are encouraging, especially for someone just starting on their journey. Sometimes I was too busy to even think about shopping, but buying online made it so easy and efficient. I now also get a weekly delivery of a box filled with organic and free-range fruit, veg and other cooking ingredients. A box by a super company called 'Mindful Chef' here in the UK gives me everything I need to make incredibly tasty and healthy meals with ease.

I stopped using the microwave and started cooking the old-fashioned way. I kept trying to think how my grandmother would have bought food, prepared it, and cooked it. I eliminated most plastic products – from polystyrene and plastic containers, to plastic cups and clingfilm. This came after discovering a study in Environmental Health Perspectives that had collated evidence to suggest that plastics can release chemicals that mimic the sex hormone estrogen.[19]

I decided to get a blood test, and hair analysis food intolerance test, to confirm the wheat intolerance and any other food sensitivities. The hair analysis test is inexpensive and can be done by sending a few pieces of hair off to a laboratory where they advise what foods you may be intolerant or allergic too. (The results of the hair analysis test matched the blood test I also instructed at the same time; although it was ten times the cost!)

You can visit your doctor in the UK and ask to be tested for wheat and gluten intolerances. Although, if you have excluded either for some time, they do not always show up. If you are unsure, just pay attention to your body symptoms after you eat. I am okay with gluten; what caused me the most excruciating pain was wheat, and this is the case for most endometriosis sufferers. However, if you find excluding wheat alone does not improve your monthly painful ordeal, then it is worth getting gluten sensitivity checked out as well.

I was advised to avoid soy products at all costs. Before this, I had no knowledge about the impact of it on my health. In fact, I do not think most people realise how hard soy is on their body. I had previously read in a magazine how women in Japan had fewer period issues because they ate a lot of soy. So, innocently, I then proceeded to consume large amounts of tofu, tubs full of soy nuts and began drinking soy milk. This resulted in the heaviest haemorrhaging of blood I had ever seen on my next monthly period. I was so shocked. I would later learn that soy is a very estrogenic product and needs to be removed from the diet. Avoid drinking soy milk (which is a popular alternative to cow's milk right now) and eating things like soy sauce and tofu. Be careful also with vegan and vegetarian products as they are often filled with soy. However, do try coconut milk, oat milk, rice milk, or even goat's milk (which my son used when he was younger) – but not soy milk.

Hypochlorhydria

I did a home test to check my stomach acid, to check for a condition called hypochlorhydria or achlorhydria. Having good stomach acid at a pH of three is essential for good health, but a lot of painkillers and pharmaceutical drugs can damage the intestinal tract, creating digestion issues. I suffered a lot of discomforts, felt heavy pressure and burning in my stomach after every meal. My GP put me on tablets to reduce acid, thinking the pain was due to excess acid, but unfortunately they made me feel worse.

I then had a gastroscopy procedure, which involved having a tube that was the thickness of my thumb inserted down my throat to inspect my oesophagus and stomach. That was a genuinely awful procedure and could have been prevented with a simple home HCL test. What I thought was heartburn and indigestion due to high stomach acid was, in fact, the complete opposite, and a symptom of stomach acid deficiency.

When the food in your stomach reaches a pH of about two to four, the valve at the bottom of the stomach (pyloric sphincter) starts to slowly release the stomach contents into the duodenum. From here, the pH goes up and down as your stomach contents travel through the intestines and out the other end. If the acid in your stomach is insufficient from the beginning, everything from the stomach to the small and large intestine will likely be compromised. Without sufficient stomach acid, your body cannot break down the food you ingest – therefore no matter what you eat, if it is not likely to be broken down or absorbed, you will not benefit from its full nutrition. Think of it like this: chewing your food is the first crucial step to perfect digestion, and stomach acid is the second most important.

How to carry out the Stomach Acid Home Test:

1. Mix 1/4 teaspoon of baking soda in 4-6 ounces of cold water first thing in the morning before eating and drinking anything.
2. Drink the complete baking soda solution.
3. Time how long it takes you to burp. Wait up to five minutes to time.

If your stomach is producing adequate amounts of stomach acid, you will likely burp immediately or within two to three minutes. Burping after three minutes indicates a low acid level. If you have not burped within five minutes, then it could be an indicator that you have little or no levels of hydrochloric acid in the stomach.

This test is a good indicator, but you may want to do more testing to confirm or try to supplement with Betaine HCL tablets on your next meal. I admit I was a little nervous about trying and supplementing with these tablets. I think the name 'acid' made me feel uneasy. Betaine hydrochloride (HCL) comes in capsule form, so they bypass the teeth (so they are not affected), and despite my initial concern I responded well and lost the pressure, bagged up, and bloated feeling after meals. I was also able to eat protein more easily, as before I had found it hard to digest these foods. The Betaine HCL also helped improve my bowel function and regularity too.

For the next few years, I excluded wheat, sugar and made the necessary adjustments to my eating habits, and it worked really well for me.

Occasionally, if I ever ate wheat (without my knowledge), I would feel immediate abdominal cramps and pain, which would then take 2-3 days to subside.

My periods became far more manageable over time, and I had no clots and less bleeding. Things seemed to be going well. I started my own residential real estate property business and engaged in socialising with friends again. Even though I still suffered from exhaustion and chronic fatigue, it was a total relief to be pain-free.

Chapter 7 -

Characteristics of An Endometriosis Woman

* * *

The difference between a successful person and others is not a lack of strength, not a lack of knowledge but rather in a lack of will

— *Vince Lombardi*

S o, how does a woman with endometriosis survive in the real

world? What are the characteristics of a woman with endometriosis?

Women with this debilitating condition can and will display some general behavioural characteristics and personality types. From my observations of myself and others, women with endometriosis are fiercely loyal, stoic, determined, strong, lifelong caregivers, and often high achievers. They invariably have robust mental constitutions (they need to endure the severity and prolonged nature of endometriosis pain) and often put other people ahead of looking after themselves. They are empathetic to the point of losing themselves; they are also incredibly thoughtful and kind. Some women with endometriosis hold highly responsible positions, which can demand a lot from them both physically, emotionally, and mentally. Many women prefer to operate from a place of control. Some of their most dominant traits or 'parts' include perfectionism, being strong people pleasers, and needing a sense of order. It has been said that women with endometriosis hold their real feelings 'deep down and within' their abdomen.

Despite being unwell and continuously suffering from pain, women with endometriosis are still able to draw upon their adrenal glands and adrenaline to push themselves forward in their lives every day. It allows them to have phenomenal energy during the times that they need to override the pain and fatigue that haunts their body. Little do they know that the continual output of cortisol from the adrenal glands will aggravate the endometriosis and inflammation even further. This is because progesterone is a precursor to cortisol (the stress hormone) so, when cortisol levels rise, progesterone levels fall – as it 'steals' from progesterone, further enhancing the hormonal imbalance of estrogen.

A hormonal imbalance can be intensified because the body, regularly, is overusing the natural 'fight or flight' mechanism, which is only designed to be used for emergencies and life-threatening situations. This characteristic, plus environmental pollutants, poor diet, nutritional deficiencies and estrogen dominance (along with low progesterone), explains why women with endometriosis find themselves experiencing chronic fatigue, exhaustion, and other autoimmune conditions. The body of a woman is not designed for all these toxins and external stressors over long periods which can sometimes stretch to decades. One very severe consequence of this action is the total shutdown of ovarian function, which promotes further estrogen dominance – the real driving force behind endometriosis.

As mentioned before, despite these looming consequences, women with endometriosis interestingly often choose careers that demand excellence, perfection, competition, long working hours, and huge responsibilities. They usually go to great lengths in their work and careers. Their work, combined with their generous caretaking of others, becomes a 'way out' or distraction from their feeling of no control over the disease. The more out of control we feel with our bodies, the more we can drive ourselves harder at work, resulting in us holding high and unrealistic expectations of ourselves and our performance, and a worsening of our condition.

This is why some personality experts call endometriosis the 'running away disease' or the 'wandering womb' – women with endometriosis run away from taking care of themselves, nurturing themselves, and embracing their natural femininity. They do this by keeping busy, by living a highly pressured lifestyle and by focusing more on their families, friends, and work, than themselves.

Many women are brought up in a culture that encourages this 'selfless' behaviour. We can feel guilty sometimes even thinking about putting ourselves ahead of another person. The truth is, this façade of a superwoman-like mentality and physical strength comes about because, as women who suffer from endometriosis, we may believe ourselves to be weakened by our disease. On a subconscious level, our frustration and determination is perhaps our driving force. Sadly, though, this can affect our relationship with our body, making us more resentful of our condition and our inability to put ourselves first. We feel we are alone and lost in this condition. This is what drives us to seek approval, acceptance, recognition, and self-worth by excelling in our performance, achievements, and capabilities – although this can cause tremendous stress.

The principle of the 'oxygen mask' rule is appropriate for women with endometriosis. On an aeroplane you will hear a flight attendant say to put on your own oxygen mask first, before helping another person. Whilst it might feel counter-intuitive to hear this, no one can help others if they have run out of oxygen and are unconscious. It is very easy for endometriosis women to be overly caring and to feel responsible for others, and therefore – in the case of this analogy – not put on their own masks first. We can end up as the caregivers, the people-pleasers, the helpers, the nurturers, and the workaholics so that we can unknowingly avoid caring for ourselves. You essentially end up helping everyone else with their masks, and forget about yourself. This is why women with endometriosis eventually get so ill.

Although our bodies are designed for short bursts of stress, prolonged periods of stress – chronic stress – can be damaging to our health. Equally, if a woman is doing a job that has no meaning or purpose for her, or is away from appreciative people, or if she feels unsafe or that she cannot trust, her stress levels will be activated and then her body will be under a lot more strain.

When a woman receives no empathy or compassion for her endometriosis pain and suffering from family, friends, or work colleagues, or there is great uncertainty in her life, stress levels will be activated further. When combined with living in a 'toxic' environment – for example, living with angry neighbours or next to a noisy, polluted road – this can significantly impact a woman's health. When the body is stressed, cortisol (the stress hormone) is released into the bloodstream, which can cause the immune system to become 'resistant' and overproduce inflammatory cytokines that further compromise the immune system.

Caregiving is a natural and maternal behaviour of most women and mothers. When she was a little girl society may have encouraged her always to consider others, and she would have mirrored her mother in taking on other people's feelings and emotions whilst denying her own.

Caregiving is a critical adaptation and essential for the needs of a developing and vulnerable child growing up. However, when caretaking becomes imbalanced and excessive to the detriment of the woman, it may make her unwell.

This imbalance may come when a woman is encouraged to devote all of her time to helping others in the family whilst simultaneously being made to feel guilty or even ashamed to take care of herself – thus leaving her feeling depleted emotionally.

Some studies have shown that caregivers have to deal with acute stressors in their daily life which can have a detrimental effect on the effectiveness of the immune system.[20] As you can read, when women are emotionally stressed and isolated, there is a greater propensity for disease and illness. The degree of illness perpetuating in our society reflects our habits, our environment, and our culture.

I was lucky enough to work with the life coach Suzy Grieve who is also the author of the books *The Big Leap* and *The Big Peace*, and the editor of *Psychologies Magazine* in the UK. Her teachings and philosophy started to open my mind to a concept she referred to as 'my relationship with my body and mind'. Ultimately, at that point, I did not have one. I had viewed my body as this vessel that carried my head around – a head that was perpetually berating, chastising and criticising me and that was wracked with a swirling pool of anxiety over everything. Suzy introduced the idea that our bodies are always trying to communicate with us, but that many of us have become disconnected from them. When we ignore our body, it then 'screams' out at us in pain.

Our busy lifestyles mean we spend less time in nature or walking or even sitting in silence, and therefore less time listening to or hearing our bodies. Also, there is so much 'white noise' and so many other distractions (like social media) that it can be hard to listen to our bodies screaming out to us. Suzy also introduced the notion of asking myself the following questions: "*Who are you at 'pains' to please?*", "*Who is 'painful' in your life?*", and "*Who drains energy from you?*"

I wonder if you have heard the story about the 'Frog in a Pot'?

If a frog is placed in a pot of hot water, it will jump out immediately to escape the danger. On the other hand, if that same frog is put into a pot of cold water, and that cold water is warmed up slowly to boiling point over time, the frog will stay and be boiled to death. The temperature is so gradual, almost imperceptible, that the frog does not realise it is boiling to death.

This was something that, unwittingly, was happening in my life at this time.

I was being 'boiled' alive by my toxic relationships, my toxic work, my toxic home-life, and toxic environment – although, at that time, I was not aware of it.

Chapter 8 -

When The 'Endometriosis Diet' Stopped Working...

* * *

What lies behind us and what lies before us, are tiny matters to
what lies within us

— Ralph Waldo Emerson

F ast forward to 2010. It was nine years since I had started

the 'endometriosis diet', but now I had ended up in the accident and emergency department of the local hospital, writhing around in excruciating pain. Although the endometriosis dietary changes, and the elimination of wheat, had initially (and for many years) made a significant reduction in my pain and improved my menstrual cycles, suddenly it was not enough. Something had gone horribly wrong, but I did not know what.

I was 43 years old when the endometriosis flare-up occurred. I had been aware of an ever-increasing amount of stress building in my work and personal life. With that, my pelvis had been feeling increasingly uncomfortable over the previous six months. I was aware of many pressures in my life at that time, and I used to remark at how they 'vampirised my soul' and made me feel like I was 'walking through treacle' every day. I was so disappointed to be back in hospital. Why had this endometriosis diet stopped working?

I was in so much agonising pain that the doctors prescribed me double doses of morphine, in addition to 36 painkillers a day. But it was to no avail – the pain maintained its throbbing and acidic intensity and absolutely nothing the doctors gave me lessened the pain. Every morning for the 15 days I was in hospital, the consultant would waltz into the ward, followed by their entourage. The consultant would look at notes on a clipboard for all of about three minutes, look down their nose at this 'body in a bed' – i.e. me – and then prescribe some other painkiller or drug. Whenever I tried to explain that I recognised my symptoms as a flare-up of endometriosis, I would be patronised and given a disdainful look. They would remark about how I could not have endometriosis as I had been able to have children, and I had not been on medications or drugs for nine years. And then the entourage would trot off again.

After a few days, when it became apparent the medications were not working, I secretly stopped taking the painkillers that the nurses kept giving me. I would wait until the nurses had gone, and then I would put them into my handbag. The drugs and painkillers were making me cloudy headed, and there was no point taking something that was not helping. It was essential for me to avoid any of their side effects too, and I needed to have a clear head. I needed to think. I needed to figure out what to do.

I was scared. The pain was intensifying and I was still in hospital after 12 days. The painkillers made no difference to the pain but were starting to cause me unpleasant side effects, like breathing difficulties and eczema. I asked to stop the morphine as it did nothing for the pain either, but made me want to vomit continuously. (I later learned that this is a common side effect and anti-sickness injections should have been given to me.) The nurses (the unsung heroes of hospitals) were wonderfully supportive and actually apologetic about the arrogance of some of the doctors and consultants. One nurse even encouraged me to keep taking the morphine so they would understand how ill I truly was. But I could not. The drugs were only adding to the problems my body was experiencing.

At this point, I was fighting two battles – one fighting endometriosis and the other fighting to be believed.

After a few more days, my head was clear of painkillers and morphine, and I insisted on speaking to the head of the gynaecological department. I managed to convince him that something was seriously wrong with me. That same afternoon, I was wheeled into the operating theatre for a diagnostic laparoscopy. Despite the fact that previous X-rays, MRI scans, abdominal scans and transvaginal ultrasound showed no signs of cysts, endometriosis or adhesions, the laparoscopy confirmed evidence of them all.

Prior to this confirmation, the doctors had been saying they could see nothing so, therefore, there must be nothing. This is a common problem for women with endometriosis. They have chronic debilitating pain, but there is no blood test to confirm the condition. Scans or X-rays rarely show anything. So instead of the medical profession believing the woman's pain, they make her feel that she is somehow a hypochondriac and 'making it up'. Even to this day, this belief persists in the minds of some medical professionals. It is already bad enough for women to suffer at all, but then to have to fight to be believed and helped can destroy the soul.

Sadly, I woke up from my surgery still in pain. The nurses shared with me, however, that the notes on my file stated they had found eight chocolate cysts as well as endometrial blood fluid in my pelvis. This 'spillage' was the cause of the pain. The hot burning blood was from one cyst which had burst and emptied its contents all over my uterus, ovaries, bowel, and bladder. No wonder I was in so much pain. However, despite the temporary satisfaction I felt from getting confirmation that I was not going mad, I soon realised that they had just opened me up, had a look around and sewn me back up! They had done nothing to try help. The surgeon had not removed any of the offending cysts or liquid. I was distraught – and still in chronic pain.

I was told I would need to be referred to another consultant and get another operation. I was discharged later that day with nothing more than painkillers. I was told I would have to wait a minimum of 12 weeks on the National Health Service (NHS) to be seen by a consultant gynaecologist. What was I to do in the meantime? No one had any answers. I was just expected to 'put up and shut up'.

My children were very distressed to see me in such agonising pain when I got home. My son and daughter both cried when they saw me almost passing out in pain on the bathroom floor repeatedly over the next few days. My husband worked away from home, so I was entirely responsible for my children, and I was on my own. I had no one to call upon – no family or friends. I tried very hard to put on a 'brave' face for my children's sake, but it was hard when the pain would come and grab me from nowhere and take my breath away. Even worse for my children, it would sometimes have me unexpectedly screaming out and doubled up in pain without warning.

My local doctor suggested going privately to speed up the process if I could afford it. If I were to use the NHS, the waiting list was 12 weeks to see the consultant, and then a further nine weeks to have the operation. A total of 21 weeks (almost five months) before I might be released from this pain. However, I emptied my savings account and went privately, which meant I was able to see a consultant and have the operation within three days!

It cost me several thousand pounds of my savings, and the following week I underwent a surgery that consisted of radical abdominal excision and cystectomy. This surgery was to remove all endometrial deposits, cysts and adhesions. I viewed it like I was a car going in for its yearly service. I envisaged I was going to be wheeled into the theatre, cut open, 'cleaned out' and sewn back up. I thought I would be back up on my feet, like new, within a few weeks.

But that never happened.

I just got progressively worse and worse.

Six weeks after the private surgery, although the acid pain had gone, I had started to develop new and disturbing symptoms and pain. I was troubled with this new deep, throbbing, contraction-like pain and pressure in my lower abdomen.

I emailed the consultant, and he reassured me, telling me to 'give it time' as it was probably the body still healing. After ten weeks, I felt no better. I was starting to get distraught. I was getting worse and worse, not better. This new pain was intensifying, and it felt like I was about to give birth at any moment. I had this 'bearing down' feeling and shooting pains up my vagina. I was terrified now. All this money had been spent, my business was in limbo, and I had no money coming in. I was unable to work or care for my children. I was in excruciating pain and had to spend most of my days in the house, bed-bound. I did not know what would become of me.

As the symptoms progressed, I emailed the consultant again and again. The consultant informed me that he thought I had now developed another condition called adenomyosis, and started talking straight away about a hysterectomy. I was horrified that he immediately spoke about a hysterectomy and did not explore other options. I insisted on getting confirmation of this new condition, but he said that only an MRI scan could do that. I decided that I would get my own MRI scan done after being told it would be another 12 weeks waiting time on NHS.

Adenomyosis can often be classified with or misinterpreted as endometriosis, and can cause severe pelvic pain and menstrual irregularities. Adenomyosis occurs when nodules or knots of endometrial tissue develop and grow into and within the smooth deep muscle layers of the uterus. Sadly, the MRI confirmed that endometriosis was still in my pelvis whilst also showing that adenomyosis was now evident too.

My Journal Extract
Friday 29th April 2011, 01.02 am

"I am sat here in the kitchen crying and sobbing. I feel so utterly depressed, lonely, alone and a total big fat failure. I feel so weak and exhausted. My tummy is in so much pain. I feel so scared and depressed. Why am I still ill? It has been over four months now. I feel there is no end in sight. What is to become of me, I wonder? Is this it? Will I be ill, in pain, shuffling around, doubled over with a hot water bottle attached to my belly, forever? House and bed-bound, a total home bird and social recluse. I am sick of making plans and having to cancel them. I am sick of making excuses to people and having to try and explain the pain. The unpredictability of endometriosis is so hard, especially when people keep saying that I look okay! It makes me want to scream. I do not want to sound like I am feeling sorry for myself, but I struggle to put a brave face on and to pretend my endometriosis is not tearing me up inside. I am finding it's easier to pretend that I am okay. I can see people thinking "is she making this up?" How on earth could you make up this pain and living nightmare!? No one could make this up. Do people genuinely think anyone would choose the existence that I have right now? That is what it feels like; 'an existence'. It is a big struggle to get through each hour, let alone each day.

I keep hoping and praying for a way out; for someone to help me. Surely there must be another way, other than the touted 'cure' referred to as a hysterectomy. A hysterectomy is no cure, but a way of getting you out of the gynaecologist's ear and putting more money in his pocket. I feel lost right now and in a dark, overgrown maze, suffocating in the cycle of the medical machine… Dear God, please help me''.

The consultant's suggestion for me to have a hysterectomy felt an extreme one. What was evident to me, however, was that once my uterus and ovaries were removed in a hysterectomy, I would no longer be referred back to the gynaecological department as all my 'gynaecological parts' would have been removed.

It felt like I was being passed along the well-worn conveyor belt of the medical machine, to be processed like a product and not a person and discarded at the end when the inevitable happened and I did not get better. More importantly, a hysterectomy is not a cure for endometriosis, and it has so many life-changing, horrific side effects, but surely the consultant knew that?

It was time to re-evaluate other options that might be available to me.

Chapter 9

Surgery Side Effects

* * *

Hope springs eternal
— Alexander Pope

I t was back to the drawing board for me. I took the time to re-

examine what had gone wrong and where I was currently. I looked again at what else the modern medical machine could offer me by way of surgical or hormone treatments, and it appeared to be a long list of invasive treatments with damaging side effects.

What I had come to realise was that surgery was not the 'quick fix' I had hoped it would be. It should have been the very last option, and I only should have considered it after I had done thorough research on the procedure to understand the risks and side effects. I should have taken more time, and made sure I had a long conversation with the surgeon.

For instance, I learned that before any surgical procedure, your abdomen is covered with an antiseptic substance (povidone-iodine) which is used to try and sterilise the incision area. This substance can be toxic to our mitochondria (which are the little energy battery packs inside our cells). When our mitochondria have toxic substances inhibiting their function, our bodies are less able to operate effectively, and chronic fatigue may develop. Then during the operation, the abdomen is inflated with carbon dioxide so the surgeon can get easier access to your abdominal organs and more space for the instruments. These two substances alone can add additional toxic stress to an already sick and pained body.

I also learned that endometriosis could cause severe inflammation in the pelvic cavity, which results in the formation of scar tissue, referred to as 'adhesions'. As mentioned previously, these adhesions are best compared in appearance to the thin white skin that can be seen atop chicken breasts. When adhesions form, they can restrict organs in the pelvic area from moving and cause them to stick together – leading to a condition referred to as a 'frozen pelvis'. And operations to help this just end up causing more adhesions.

Endometriosis can grow into the layers of tissue in your organs and interfere with the nerve endings. You may experience what appears to be unrelated pain, but it can radiate into the back, legs and vulva. Tissues and cysts may fill with liquid, which spills out over the organs and causes irritation, chronic and acute pain. On top of this, operations also irritate other nerve endings and organs.

When our body has an injury of any kind, prostaglandins are released into the area to attack the offending 'enemy', by activating an inflammatory response. This process perpetuates the prolonged and continued agonising pain that women with endometriosis experience. Inflammatory issues remain a problem after any operation and, if anything, are aggravated by it.

Let us look at the range of invasive operations that are currently offered to women with endometriosis:

Diagnostic Laparoscopy

A diagnostic laparoscopy is used to confirm a suspected diagnosis of endometriosis and to evaluate the severity of the condition. During the laparoscopy operation, the surgeon determines the number, size, and location of endometrial implants and adhesions (if they can be seen). In theory, the surgeon is expected to drain any cysts, cut, burn, or separate any adhesions, but this does not always happen. Some surgeons merely confirm 'diagnosis' of endometriosis implants and then finish the operation without the removal of endometrial implants.

The keyhole surgical procedure involves a small incision in the abdomen and the insertion of a small thin fibre-optic tube with a valve called a laparoscope. The laparoscope is equipped with a tiny telescopic lens, which enables the doctor to view the uterus, ovaries, tubes, and peritoneum (lining of the pelvis) on a video monitor.

Although laparoscopy is regarded as a conservative surgery, the side effects and risks are many and undertaking any operation should be taken seriously. The lasers that are expected to burn or cut adhesions can sometimes hit the bladder, bowel, uterus, ovaries, fallopian tubes, and abdominal wall, causing severe long term side effects.

Another significant issue is the reoccurrence of adhesions and cysts soon after the surgery. As the body has been cut open and the internal organs moved about, cut, and burnt, then the inflammatory and repair process in the body begins again. This means adhesions that have just been cut may regrow due to the body's natural need to want to repair. The vicious cycle of operation, adhesions, operation, adhesions continues. Put simply: endometriosis causes adhesions and operations cause adhesions so an operation to help endometriosis and adhesions is going to make the situation worse.

I read about a woman who had 26 operations for her endometriosis, and not only did it not prevent the return of her endometriosis but it made her worse, and she became sicker and sicker with each surgery. An operation is a very damaging invasion to a body that is already under chronic stress and inflammation.

Laparotomy

A laparotomy is an operation where the surgeon makes a large incision into the abdomen. In some cases, if complications occur and a large access site is needed for the surgeon, a laparoscopy can turn into a laparotomy.

Laparoscopy Ablation and Excision

An ablation and excision laparoscopic operation is when the surgeon spends longer removing, scraping and cutting out the endometrial deposits, lesions, cysts or adhesions that can be seen. However, the operation does not prevent or limit the recurrence of lesions and symptoms. The operation is a traumatic experience for the body, and the reoccurrence of adhesions may occur within weeks. In addition, there may be long-term bladder or bowel injury or ovarian dysfunction.

Pre-Sacral-Neurectomy (PSN)

Pre-sacral-neurectomy is a procedure where the surgeon cuts the nerves that transmit the pain from your uterus to your brain. The surgeon has to cut through numerous blood vessels. Evidence suggests that PSN carries a high risk, is incomplete and is subject to controversy.

Laparoscopic Uterine Nerve Ablation (LUNA)

Laparoscopic uterine nerve ablation is when the surgeon cuts the sympathetic and para-sympathetic uterosacral nerves that transmit pain from the uterus to the brain. Evidence suggests that LUNA carries a high risk and is incomplete. Just like PSN, LUNA is subject to controversy.

Da Vinci Surgical System

The da Vinci Surgical System is a robotic technology conducted by a surgeon manipulating robotic arms within the woman's abdomen. While robotic surgery is considered generally safe, the Food and Drug Administration (FDA) in the United States is reviewing this after a growing number of reports of related complications. The side effects can be devastating, and there may be life-altering injuries including burns, tears and other problems in the abdomen and surrounding tissues. For example, one woman, after undergoing surgery by the da Vinci Surgical System, found her ureter to be burned and colon damaged.[21] This is only one of the over 20,000 adverse robot-related events that have been reported to the FDA.

Many people miss the point. Whilst the robot may be more precise in some aspects, the surgeon in control is still a human and, therefore, still very much able to make errors. More significantly, the patient is undergoing surgery so, regardless of what or who is doing your surgery, your body is being cut open and invaded, and thus will be subject to the inevitable surgical aftereffects like adhesions and inflammation.

I felt I had reached a dead-end, a no-through road. What was I to do? I was still in excruciating pain. I was unable to leave the house, play with my children, go to work, and my old clients had moved on to my competitors.

Many, if not all, of the medical treatment options being suggested to me felt barbaric and had awful side effects. I had spent thousands of pounds trying the laparoscopy ablation and excision surgery route, but it had failed me. The surgeon had assured me that all of the adhesions, cysts and endometrial deposits would be removed and I would be back on my feet in no time. Yet here I was in a worsened condition within weeks of the operation, not better. What on earth was going on in my body?

I found myself wrestling back and forth endlessly with my old beliefs that the medical profession was my only option, and that they had to 'fix' me.

However, I realised that to the 'medical machine' I was just a number, a body in a bed and someone to process. The options I was being given did not feel like options at all, merely a life sentence to dependency on painkillers, hormonal drugs, and surgery. That did not feel like life for me.

Chapter 10 -

The Hysterectomy Hoax

* * *

God grant me the serenity to accept the things I cannot change,
the courage to change the things I can, and the wisdom to know
the difference

– Serenity Prayer

I n 1999, a study found that an estimated 20 million women in the USA have had a hysterectomy operation performed. Twenty years later, that figure is likely to be many millions higher, given that our environment has grown to be even more toxic, and the number of women in the world has also increased. By the age of 60 years old, roughly a third of all women will have had a hysterectomy. Hysterectomy is the second most frequently performed surgical procedure with around 600,000 operations carried out in the USA each year.[22] As you can see, endometriosis is a BIG issue and hysterectomies are an even BIGGER business.

After a woman with endometriosis reaches a certain age or has had children, the most common suggestion by doctors is to have a hysterectomy. Yet very few women question the validity and necessity of this procedure. Your uterus is more than just a 'baby bag', as some doctors like to refer to it. A hysterectomy operation involves the removal of a woman's sex organs (the equivalent is removing a man's testicles and penis) – it is female castration, and causes lifelong damage to the body.

In his fascinating book, '*The Hysterectomy Hoax*', Dr Stephen West says that only 2% of hysterectomies are warranted, and generally only in the case of cancer. The uterus is a vital organ and, even though it does not directly produce hormones, its removal is enough to cause hormone imbalances. Some of these hormones help to prevent the development of conditions like heart disease and osteoporosis (thinning of the bones). As mentioned previously, a hysterectomy will also cause structural damage to your body as the uterus helps to support the pelvic bones, bladder, and bowel. A hysterectomy is NOT a cure for endometriosis, as any endometrial lesions or deposits that were in the abdominal cavity may still be there after the uterus has been removed.

Nora W. Coffey set up the *Hysterectomy Education Resources and Services (HERS) Foundation* and is the author of the enlightening book called '*The H Word*'. Her book offers real-life stories of the horrors that women have faced after hysterectomy surgeries and the untold damage to a woman's self-esteem. Nora's *HERS Foundation* is an excellent resource if you are seeking further advice and provides free information if you feel pressure to have or are considering a hysterectomy. Nora has gathered evidence for over ten years about the horrendous side effects of having a hysterectomy, and she has recorded over 150 different side effects from over 1000 women who underwent a hysterectomy.[23]

I was very fortunate to speak with Nora personally during this unsettled time, and she informed me about all the risks. It was pretty hard to ignore them and go blindly on. I knew I had to slow down and stop being reactive and do some further research.

It became clear to me that despite the mounting pressure from my partner and many doctors and surgeons to have a hysterectomy, this procedure was not an option for me because of how it had failed my mother decades before.

Although one day I almost did relent, and felt tempted to proceed down that pathway. The pain had become increasingly unbearable. I was sobbing and distraught, desperate for a way out. I could not take the pain any more. In an impulsive moment, I tried to call the hospital to arrange the hysterectomy. I did not want one, but I felt there were no other options being presented to me.

The telephone number rang and rang until finally it rang out. This was a telephone that was usually answered immediately by an efficient team of secretaries. Fortunately for me that day it was not answered when I called.

An hour later I received a telephone call from Dian Shepperson Mills, the nutritionist and author of the book '*Endometriosis: A Guide to Healing Through Nutrition*'. I had been trying to contact her for a few days, and as soon as I explained my situation, she reassured me to hold firm *"Do not let them remove your uterus Wendy!"* she said. Dian reiterated the permanent damage a hysterectomy operation causes a woman, how every woman needs their uterus long after child baring years and reminded me that the operation wouldn't cure a few areas of your life.

My mother was never the same after her operation and talked of her great regret in having a hysterectomy carried out. I shall be forever grateful to Dian for telephoning me back that day and saving my uterus and my life.

A hysterectomy may appear an attractive solution, and a super quick fix, but it is not. If it were that simple, then endometriosis would no longer be such a severe condition to have, and far fewer women would suffer from it. The many severe side effects are rarely explained to women. Equally, women who have had a hysterectomy invariably fail to realise that the onset of new symptoms and problems they experience afterwards is due to the removal of their vital sex organs.

Sadly, there is little or no support for a woman once her female organs have been removed and the gynaecological department has closed its file on her. She is never referred back to that department as she has no gynaecological 'parts' left, so is invariably passed around various departments in the process of trying to establish the source of new signs and symptoms.

After learning about the uterus's important structure and positioning in the body, I realised why a hysterectomy would cause new symptoms:

Uterus – The Heart of the South

The uterus (or womb) is situated in the heart of the pelvis and is often referred to as the 'heart of the south'. It is positioned in between the bladder and intestines (and keeps them separate). The removal of the uterus displaces these organs. Consider a carefully designed architectural structure; if the central part is removed, the surrounding areas will all shift and move. The three sets of ligaments that are cut during surgery are designed to hold the uterus in place and connect it to the cervix, floor and walls of the pelvis. These ligaments contain nerve endings which are sensitive to movement and play a role in pelvic pain if contorted by adhesions.

The uterus is best known as the organ where a baby grows, and unfortunately many doctors only view the organ for this purpose; sometimes referring to the uterus as a 'baby bag'. The lining of the uterus is called the endometrium and provides nourishment for a growing baby. At the bottom of the uterus is the cervix, which is a passage that leads to the vagina, allowing for expulsion of menstrual flow and intake of sperm. When endometriosis is on the cervix, it can cause pain on contact and tenderness. During sex, when the penis enters the vagina, it often contacts the cervix which causes pain or discomfort during sex, and then in some cases bleeding.

Some doctors fail to realise the significance and importance of female sex organs, and often suggest the removal of them through a hysterectomy as a 'cure'. However, without a uterus, a woman will not be able to experience a female uterine orgasm. This is the equivalent of a man having his penis and testicles removed. A hysterectomy causes damage to the vagina and can result in the development of symptoms like urinary incontinence, bone thinning, and weight gain. There is also evidence to suggest that women under the age of 35 who have undergone a hysterectomy are at a 4.6-fold greater risk of congestive heart failure and a 2.5-fold greater risk of coronary artery disease.[24]

It is worth repeating that a hysterectomy is NOT a cure for endometriosis. Some doctors, consultants and gynaecologists may make having the 'troublesome' organ removed sound a simple solution or sensible idea but do not be fooled. Unless you address the root causes of the endometriosis, pain, and symptoms, it may all return as it did for my mother. Any endometriosis lesions in the abdomen not seen or removed during the surgery will continue to grow, shed, and bleed in response to estrogen in the body. Be sure to do all your own extensive research and stand firm if you feel pressurised into this course of action. A hysterectomy may cause lifelong damage to a woman's body.

Nora Covey's own story is quite harrowing. She was strapped down to a hospital bed and forced against her will to have a hysterectomy. She was devastated by the events and has since made it her mission to share the untold horrors such surgery can bring. One particular part of her story still sticks in my head even now. She mentioned in her book 'The H Word' how after the removal of her uterus and ovaries she struggled to swim 'normally'. A keen swimmer beforehand, her body was now unable to float in the swimming pool and she noticed her body now tilted to the side. As you can read, your uterus is an essential organ and one worth holding on to, for many reasons.

Ovaries

One oval-shaped ovary about the size of a large grape is positioned on either side of the uterus and is attached to fallopian tubes which lead to the uterus. The ovaries are responsible for the production of estrogen and progesterone. These two primary female hormones are principally involved in the woman's maturation of the reproductive system and cyclic changes in the endometrium. The surgical removal of ovaries (oophorectomy or ovariectomy) along with the uterus results in the women being thrown into immediate menopause, which can be very severe. Side effects can include hot flushes, osteoporosis, and depression, to name a few. The rate of complications and side effects are high, with women who get their ovaries removed experiencing a significantly higher risk of mortality than those who do not.[25]

The Bladder

The bladder is a very sensitive organ that is positioned above the uterus. The urethra is a small tube that connects the kidneys to the bladder. Sometimes, due to adhesions and endometriosis deposits, the tube can become bent or tangled, which in turn causes referred pain in the kidneys, situated in the lower back region. Pressure and urgency to pee can be triggered when there is either too much inflammation in the body, if there is an overconsumption of sugar, or if endometriosis lesions are attached to the bladder. Many women experience an increase in discomfort in their bladder and increased infections after a hysterectomy. This may be because the surgeon has grazed or aggravated the bladder or bowel with their tools during the operation, or because the bladder now sits on top of the bowel, when the uterus had previously separated them. Some women may lose all bladder sensation for days or longer after surgery and require a catheter to be fitted. This can be particularly distressing for women whose bladder sensation never returns. The cutting of nerve endings and ligaments also causes more trauma and sensitivity to the bladder and bowel.

The Bowel

Another organ that endometriosis tissue can implant itself onto is the bowel (also referred to as the intestines). The bowel is a long, muscular tube that is part of your digestive tract. The bowel extends from the low end of your stomach, down the small intestine into the large intestine, towards your back passage (anus). A high percentage of women with endometriosis suffer from bowel symptoms or irritable bowel syndrome (IBS). Bowel symptoms can include, but are not limited to: pain during bowel movements, changes in stool colour, blood in stools, constipation, or diarrhoea. Adhesions can wrap around the bowel, and if the surgeon makes contact with the bowel or 'nicks' it during surgery, the bowel can become affected, and sensitivity may be increased.

According to Nora, many side effects of hysterectomies are irreversible and cause lifelong damage. I know this was the case with my mother. The surgery was one of many, and she claimed to suffer post-traumatic stress disorder and profound shock afterwards. Nora Covey and Dian Shepperson Mills reminded me regularly during this time to take my time and do my research and not succumb to any external pressure. They also reassured me as my impatience increased and advised of the consequences as I wrestled on how to move forward. They reiterated to me how a hysterectomy might cause bladder incontinence as the uterus, which had previously sat in-between the bladder and bowel, would now be gone. Also, the surgery would inevitably lose the ability for a uterine orgasm as you cannot have an orgasm if there is no uterus.

They also educated me on how, during the operation, the vagina is cut and shortened when the cervix and uterus are removed. The top of the vagina is sewn up, theoretically turning the vagina into a 'pocket' which may then prolapse (i.e. turn inside out). Once the uterus and ovaries are removed, the body is then thrown into immediate menopause. Although there would be no menstrual bleeding, any endometriosis left in my body would still grow. Ovaries, following a oophorectomy or ovariectomy, experience reduced blood supply due to the cutting of blood vessels and can be damaged. As such, there is an increased risk of early ovarian failure following a hysterectomy.[26]

I realised that although I was impatient to get well, having a hysterectomy was like jumping from a chip pan into a fire. My mother had been given a hysterectomy, and she was never the same afterwards.

All this information was sobering, to say the least, and I saw there was no quick-fix medical option to help me with my endometriosis and adenomyosis. I eventually recognised that by having a hysterectomy or taking any drugs prescribed, I would merely be swapping one set of problems and symptoms for another.

Once my important female organs were removed, it was permanent. There would not be an option to get them replaced in the future with a transplant. When they were gone, they were gone, and I would be forced to live with the consequences.

Despite my frustration and impatience, I realised that a hysterectomy was not an option or route that I could take. To do so, I could potentially double, if not triple, my pain and symptoms, whilst also picking up many new side effects.

There had to be another way.

Chapter 11 -

Harmful Effects of Estrogen Dominance

* * *

Our deepest fear is not that we are inadequate. Our deepest fear is we are powerful beyond measure.

– Marianne Williamson

S andra works full-time while raising three young children, and she has been suffering from insomnia and night sweats even though she is only in her early thirties and far away from entering into menopause. Kathryn, a busy stockbroker, has such heavy periods that she is often locked in her house for seven days every month, using the excuse of 'working from home'. Patricia, newly married with an exciting job, is losing her hair, gaining weight around the middle, and always feeling exhausted. All three women are suffering from a common condition called estrogen dominance.

Nowadays, we are seeing girls reaching puberty as early as age eight. You go and ask any woman and chances are she is bound to say she has experienced premenstrual syndrome (PMS) at some time in her life, and maybe even endometriosis, fibroids, or ovarian cysts. It is rare to find a woman who does not have pain with her period. When women are told that 'pain with a period is not normal', may women are shocked. The common culprit in these conditions? Too much estrogen.

Every woman's body contains two main sex hormones: estrogen and progesterone. Estrogen is the female sex hormone and its counterpart in males is testosterone. Both hormones are present in both sexes. There are three major forms of physiological estrogens in females – estrone, estradiol, and estriol. In a woman's body, estrogen is produced mainly by the ovaries, but also in small amounts by fat cells and the adrenal cortex.

So what can trigger estrogen dominance?

- Eating non-organic foods which contain pesticides, fertilisers, hormones, and antibiotics

- Lifestyle habits like drugs (medical and recreational), smoking, alcohol, sugar, and 'junk' food

- Genetics

- Poor liver function – the liver is responsible for eliminating metabolised estrogen

- Digestive issues – these can interfere with the liver's estrogen detoxification process, leading to cortisol production which blocks progesterone receptors

- Chronic stress – this causes cortisol production

- Unresolved emotional issues

- Use of synthetic estrogens like birth control pills and hormone replacement therapy (HRT)

- Exposure to xenoestrogens found in consumer products – chemicals like BPA and SLS

I will cover these points in greater detail in the next chapter.

What is the role that estrogen plays in our bodies then? In women, estrogen plays an essential role in the growth and development of female secondary sexual characteristics such as breasts, armpit and pubic hair, endometrium, regulation of the reproductive system and the menstrual cycle. Every menstrual cycle, estrogen produces an environment suitable for fertilisation, implantation, and nutrition of the embryo. Estrogen is a crucial component in a woman's menstrual cycle and in her ability to bear children. I will show below how estrogen affects the vital organs of the female reproductive system.

In males, estrogen also plays an indispensable role in normal male reproduction, and assists in the maturation of the sperm cells. Pubertal development in boys, such as growing long bones, is attributed to the actions of androgens. However, it is now recognised as being mediated in part by estrogen.

Here is a more detailed list of estrogen's role:

Ovaries – estrogen mainly helps stimulate the growth of the egg follicle.

Vagina – estrogen stimulates the growth of the vagina to its adult size. Estrogen also thickens the vaginal wall and increases vaginal acidity to reduce the risk of bacterial infections.

Fallopian tubes – estrogen, and in particular estradiol, in particular plays a fundamental role in regulating the cell homeostasis through the estrogen receptors and ensuring the structor of the tubes.

Uterus – estrogen regulates the flow and thickness of the endometrium, the mucous membrane that lines the insides of the uterus, (while progesterone maintains the endometrium to help ensure the full term of pregnancy). Estrogen is responsible for increasing the endometrium's size and weight, the number of cells, types of cells, the flow of blood, protein content, and enzyme activity. Estrogen is also responsible for stimulating the muscles in the uterus to develop and contract. These contractions are vital as they help the uterine wall to cast off dead tissue during menstruation, and allow the delivery of a child.

Cervix – estrogen regulates the flow and thickness in the uterine mucous secretions to enhance the transport of the sperm cells.

Mammary glands – estrogen unifies with other hormones in the development of female breasts. It is responsible for the growth of the female breasts during adolescence, and the pigmentation of the nipples.

Let us delve further into the process by which estrogen plays its role during a menstrual cycle. Estrogen controls the menstrual cycle, and the amount of it in a woman's body naturally rises and falls throughout the month.

Day 1 of the cycle
Estrogen and progesterone levels at this point in the cycle are at their lowest.

Day 5 of the cycle

An egg is selected. Inside the ovary, the egg is contained within a follicle – the anatomic structure where the egg develops. The follicle will begin to release increasing amounts of estrogen.

Days 6 to 13 of the cycle

Preparing for ovulation. From this point and towards the end of this stage, estrogen levels will initially rise slowly and then will increase more rapidly.

Day 14 of the cycle

The follicle that contains the egg will break open, and the ovary will release the egg into the fallopian tube. It will stay there and wait for sperm to fertilise it. The follicle will remain in the fallopian tube.

Days 15 to 28 of the cycle

After ovulation. At this stage, the levels of progesterone will start to increase. If the egg waiting in the fallopian tube is not fertilised, both estrogen and progesterone levels will drop after two weeks, and the lining of the insides of the uterus gets ready to be shed. At this point, menstruation begins, and the cycle will start all over again.

Our menstrual cycle is a very dynamic process that repeats itself every 28 days on average, and you can see that estrogen plays a role that is important to the whole process. We endometriosis women are all too familiar with mood changes and disturbances during our periods, and estrogen is thought to be involved.

If estrogen is good for our body, why is it damaging to have too much of it? When that ratio of progesterone and estrogen is skewed, and a woman's body becomes deficient in progesterone or excessive in estrogen, either way the woman goes to a state of 'estrogen dominance'. Apart from reproduction, estrogen influences many of the other physiological processes in a woman's body, such as cardiovascular health, bone integrity, cognition, and behaviour. With this expansive role, it is not surprising that estrogen is also implicated in the development or progression of numerous diseases like cancer. This is the reason why we women should always keep estrogen levels in check.

Among the diseases that excess estrogen is linked to are: breast cancer, ovarian cancer, colorectal cancer, heart disease, neurodegenerative diseases, Alzheimer's disease, Parkinson's disease, gallstones, osteoporosis, systemic supus erythematosus (SLE), and our primary concern, endometriosis which, left unchecked, can potentially lead to endometrial cancer. Estrogen dominance can also lead to weight gain, thyroid issues, faulty blood sugar levels, depression, and blood clots.

How do we know if we are in a state of estrogen dominance?

Here is a list of common symptoms to watch out for in estrogen dominance and endometriosis:

- Unusually painful periods, heavy bleeding, or clots
- Chronic pelvic pain in lower abdomen
- Sore, swollen, tender breasts and nipples
- Irregular periods or exceptionally long periods
- Premenstrual syndrome (PMS) or premenstrual tension (PMT)
- Ovarian cysts, 'chocolate' cysts or endometriomas
- Fibroids
- Polycystic ovary syndrome (PCOS)
- Abnormal pap smear

- Migraines and head fog
- Fat gain around hips, stomach, and thighs
- Water retention
- Puffiness
- Bloating
- Hair thinning and hair loss
- Chronic fatigue
- Insomnia
- Hot flashes, burning up and night sweats
- Restless legs at night
- Excessively weepy close to your cycle
- Low thyroid function
- Lower back pain
- Painful bowel movements
- Bladder pressure and frequency of urination

If you are experiencing two or more of the above symptoms, then you may have a hormonal imbalance and in an estrogen dominance state.

Extreme cases of estrogen dominance can also be seen when there are symptoms like:

- Adenomyosis
- Uterine cancer
- Ovarian cancer
- Breast cancer

I admit to knowing very little about how my body functioned when I first started this journey, and even less about my hormonal cycle at this time. I had heard about progesterone and estrogen but was unaware of how an imbalance could have such an impact on our bodies.

'Estrogen dominance' was a phrase that I could finally identify with.

I was finally starting to understand why, despite having removed wheat and sugar from my diet, I was still in pain.

I had a severe hormonal imbalance that needed to be looked at in much greater detail.

Chapter 12 -

Our Toxic World

* * *

A journey of a thousand miles begins with a single step
                                                    – Confucius

My research led me to understand the term 'estrogen-dominance' better and also taught me that endometriosis and adenomyosis were estrogen dominant conditions. If we already have enough estrogen produced in our body, why do we still get more, and why does it cause estrogen dominance? I have touched on it briefly above, but I will cover it in more detail now.

Most women out there may not be aware of the everyday reality of poisons in our environment that have an impact on our bodies, and I think this is the right time to let you know. This was a wakeup call for me and also a turning point in my healing.

Chemicals

Every day of our lives, environmental estrogens bombard us, and we are blind to it. They are called 'xenoestrogens' or estrogen mimickers. These fabricated estrogen chemicals are imposters acting precisely like the estrogen in our bodies. These estrogen mimickers are found in almost everything, from plastics, chemicals in cosmetics, pesticides, washing powders, dry cleaning chemicals, the pollution in our environment, even food and dairy products, and so much more. If we regularly expose ourselves to all of these, we will be susceptible to additional estrogen absorption, and too much estrogen will upset the body's delicate balance of hormones.

Medications

Medications such as birth control pills or oral contraceptives and intrauterine devices like coils also contribute to estrogen dominance. Birth control pills prevent the ovulation of the egg cell, and as I described above, estrogen plays a lead role in ovulation. Therefore, if ovulation is restricted, it leaves estrogen with nothing else to do but increase in levels, and this is not good. If you do not ovulate, you do not produce progesterone as you would do if you released an egg every month. Over time, no ovulation may create a severe progesterone deficiency. Although there are many medical, social, and emotional reasons why women take birth control pills, it might be a good time to reconsider using other forms of contraceptive. This includes condoms or femidoms, or fertility awareness-based methods (FAMs) which are ways to track ovulation in order to prevent pregnancy.

Xenoestrogens

Some synthetic chemicals mimic and disrupt the hormonal balance in women. They do this by blocking or binding receptors, and because they are not biodegradable, they get stored in our fat cells. The rise in estrogen mimickers may be why there are many young girls entering puberty prematurely and why some women produce too much estrogen and too little progesterone. It could also be responsible for the 50% decrease in men's sperm count in some areas of the globe.[27]

Further confirmation of the effect of xenoestrogens was provided in a study of fish exposed to estrogenic water. In the study, researchers found that when comparing the fish exposed to estrogenic water downstream and those in normal water further upstream, the downstream fish population had half the number of males than that of the upstream population. What is more, around 20% of the downstream fish were intersex, whereas the upstream fish population had no intersex fish. This goes to show the impact of estrogen on hormone levels.[28]

Studies have shown that tap drinking water has been found to contain a primary estrogen compound that is in birth control pills called ethinylestradiol (EE), so consider getting a house water filter or drink mineral water.

One particularly harmful chemical is called glyphosate, which is used as a herbicide. Glyphosate has been shown by France's University of Caen to cause potential fertility problems, miscarriages, and premature births.[29]

Processed Food

Processed foods are also full of excess estrogens that our body does not need. Other sources of estrogen that we may unknowingly take are beef, chicken and other meats that are raised and fed with antibiotics and growth hormones. Always go organic, free-range, and fresh for your choices of food as much as possible. Then there is soy, which, by nature, already contains plant-based estrogens, referred to as 'phytoestrogens'.

Genetically Modified Food

Genetically modified foods (GMO) first came on the market in 1994 with soybean, corn, canola, cottonseed oil, sugar, and aspartame being some of the top products. Although GMOs were designed to be resistant to bugs, disease and drought and to have a longer shelf life, they have been shown to cause harm to humans and animals, with symptoms such as estrogen dysregulation. It is hard to avoid GMOs nowadays as they are in so many products. In Canada, for example, over 75% of processed foods contain at least one genetically modified ingredient.[30]

Lifestyle Habits

Too much alcohol, coffee, and artificial sugars can also contribute to estrogen dominance in our bodies. Alcohol, for one, can weaken our liver as it is a poison to the body. As we all know, our liver is our body's filter and is the key for detoxification, especially with excess hormones.

When we do not eat a well-balanced green and leafy diet with adequate protein and take on too much of one thing (such as fats, sugars, or alcohol), this makes our liver sluggish and congested, and unable to function fast enough to eliminate these toxins. Once that happens, the hormones will be left unchecked, and this will create a hormonal imbalance.

I had not realised just how toxic and poisonous our environment was. I felt irritated that I had been so trusting of global brand name products and had never even thought to question what was put in my body, on my body, or around my body. If so many of these personal care and household products were so toxic, then why were we not adequately informed that putting them in our bodies could make us so ill?

I now wanted to know what I could do to remove these toxins from my life, so a new phase of the journey began.

Chapter 13 -

Fighting Against the Toxins

* * *

Courage is not the absence of fear, but rather the judgment that
something else is more important than fear
— Ambrose Redmoon

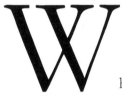hat are the ways to fight against the environmental

toxins, rebalance your hormones, and prevent estrogen dominance?

Firstly, the liver, thyroid, and adrenal glands must operate at peak performance to ensure proper hormonal balance and harmony within the body. The best way to achieve this is to employ a healthful nutrition program and to eliminate any toxins that are poisoning your body.

The liver is the largest internal organ inside the body and is considered the second largest organ to the skin. The liver is a vital organ and has many functions, but the main one is to expel toxins that are ingested into the body. The long term use of pain killers is toxic to the liver and may harm its ability to rid the body of excess estrogens.

Hormone-Free Food

Our great, great ancestors would eat cleanly and freshly from the plains and countryside. Meat was a staple part of their diet. The animals were allowed to roam and eat off the land and were not like the animals now which kept in cramped and inhumane conditions. Some women with endometriosis passionately advise others not to eat meat. Yet I believe that as long as the meat is hormone-free, free-range, and organic, then we are okay to eat meat. So consider eating only organic, grass-fed, hormone-free, free-range meat and poultry as much as possible. Try to get hold of meat from wild and free-range livestock to obtain the best lean protein.

If you are vegan, then this does not apply to you but do make sure you are consuming enough protein every day to assist your body's repair functions – but avoid soy at all costs. Also avoid dairy, artificial sugar, vegetable oils, refined flours, and refined, simple carbohydrates which may be full of E numbers, additives and preservatives – you just have to read the long list of ingredients to see what toxins your body is processing every day.

No Wheat

One type of food to remove from your diet, as I have pointed out in previous chapters, is wheat. A sign that your body has a wheat intolerance can be if you find your stomach gets bloated and distended after eating it. This is because wheat can be very hard on the digestive tract. Try an exclusion diet for three months and then reintroduce it to see the effects. Eat plenty of fibre-rich vegetables and focus primarily on the cruciferous ones like kale, broccoli, cauliflower, cabbage, pak choy, and brussels sprouts, to name a few. Broccoli comes highly recommended because it contains indole-3-carbinol (I3C), which helps in detoxifying estrogen out of the body.

No Coffee

Consider reducing and then eliminating coffee from your diet. Caffeine, a stimulant found in abundance in coffee, has been associated with an increase in estrogen in those who drink just two cups (200mg of caffeine) of coffee a day.[31] I used to be a regular consumer of thick black coffee so it was a challenge to start with. However, I over a period of a few weeks I slowly reduced the number of cups per day and then diluted it to the point it was easy to avoid. Interestingly I noticed when I stopped drinking coffee I had more energy and my body felt less wired and tired. Try a delicious alternative called rooibos (meaning 'red bush') tea instead. It is naturally caffeine-free and delicious.

No Plastics or Microwavable Packets

Avoid using the microwave or heating food in plastic materials and consider replacing any plastic kettles with stainless steel ones. A study showed that plastic cling film or wrap that is heated in a microwave has 500,000 times the minimum amount of xenoestrogens needed to stimulate and grow breast cancer cells in a test tube.[32] Quite shocking figures!

Personal Products & Cosmetics

Clean up your environment. Please get rid of all the unnecessary cosmetics, especially those with ingredients that you cannot pronounce as that is a sign it is not natural. Minimise, if not stop, applying lotions on your skin even if only temporarily, whilst you are unwell and in chronic pain. These contain xenoestrogens, parabens, and sodium laurel sulphates (SLS) which are toxic chemicals which your skin will absorb directly into the bloodstream.

Cheap brands tend to have more chemicals in them, so it is best to avoid them. One natural, and inexpensive approach I have tried and still use today, is to use coconut oil, rice bran oil, and shea butter. They give the same effect of smoothing your skin, but best of all, they are 100% natural. A lot of creams have these natural products as bases and then load the chemicals on top. Do not be fooled by the labels and claims on the front – always read the full ingredient list on the back of the product. Use organic, perfume-free, fragrance-free shampoos, conditioners, and soap bars. Avoid nail varnish and nail polish removers as they are highly toxic. Use natural paraben-free sunscreen lotions. I like using olive oil in low SPF conditions, which gives my skin a lovely colour.

Tampons

Only use organic tampons. Many tampons and sanitary pads have bleach in them, which can cause allergic toxic reactions. Toxic Shock Syndrome (TSS) is a rare but severe and sometimes fatal disease, where the body's response to the poisons (the bacteria called Staphylococcus Aureus or Staph) is to go into shock. This can be seen to affect those who use super-absorbent tampons. Never leave tampons in for more than three hours and NEVER overnight. Why not try a 'Mooncup', which is a reusable menstrual cup about two inches long. It is greener, safer, and cheaper than the chemically laden tampons or sanitary towels. Worn internally, the Mooncup catches the menstrual fluid, is leak-free, and can be worn for hours.

Household Products

For your cleaning around the house, consider using greener cleaning products, or better yet, make your own. There are hundreds of 'do-it-yourself' cleaning product recipes, and you can find them on the internet. Most of them use simple ingredients like bicarbonate of soda and vinegar that can be found already in your home. It is essential to change your washing powder, as clothes washed in chemical-laden products continue to release these chemicals when worn. Swap out with coconut-based products. There are many suppliers online which offer a vast selection, and many deliver worldwide. Do not use fabric softeners or tumble dryer sheets, as petrochemicals are used in them, and they will be directly absorbed into your skin.

Water Filter

Invest in a good quality water filter for the house, or a water filter jug. The consumption of birth control pills and other synthetic hormones contribute to estrogen contaminating the streams, rivers, and waterway systems. Try to drink water from glass bottles only, and if a plastic water container has been heated up, do NOT drink the water – instead throw it away immediately.

Detox

Detoxify your liver at least twice a year. I was able to achieve this by eating nothing but fresh free-range food for a month, practising regular vegetable juicing, and using Chlorella cracked cell powder and Spirulina. When doing a gentle detox, I can observe the positive effects because of the resulting light and energetic feeling I get afterwards. However, a word of caution: women with endometriosis need to get out of pain first and have enough energy before they can consider doing a detox. Detoxing is exhausting on the body the first few times it is done. Your body needs to be strong and have enough additional energy for the process. Remember, we are going to be healing gently, so go very slowly before thinking about doing this.

Regular Bowel Movements

Try as much as possible to practice regular bowel movements. After your liver detoxifies, it sends all the excess estrogen hormones to the stool to be excreted from your body as you poop. You are looking to discharge waste matter from the large intestine and out of the body at least once a day.

If by some misfortune you are constipated, the stool becomes immobile and the estrogens and other toxins in it can be reabsorbed through the intestines and back into your system. You do not want that. Therefore, to facilitate proper detoxification, drink a minimum of eight glasses of fresh, still (not sparkling) mineral water a day and ensure you eat organic vegetables full of fibre to keep your bowel movements regular.

Sleep

Getting a good night's sleep is easier said than done for women with endometriosis. For me, more often than not, nighttime was when the pain would escalate. If you find yourself having difficulty getting to sleep, try listening to relaxation, meditation, or mindfulness music. If that does not work then consider taking a natural sleeping aid containing melatonin, hops, chamomile, valerian, and passionflower. This worked wonders sometimes and helped me a lot. If you are finding it hard to sleep due to the pain, lie with your feet elevated, eyes closed, and focus on your breathing, which will help to get your body into a restful and healing state.

I used to get quite stressed when I was not able to sleep, but I learnt that lying down and listening to 'bilateral' or relaxing music helped me to focus on my breath, enabling my body to get into a healing state. Your overworked adrenal glands need the sleep, but even deep rest through relaxation can help assist the body to repair. When your body releases adrenaline after bouts of chronic pain or stress, you may feel exhaustion quickly once the effects of the hormone fade out. You can reverse this by getting a solid night's sleep or deep, restful periods amounting to at least eight hours a day.

Thyroid

Keep your thyroid glands healthy. Both the adrenal glands and thyroid glands are directly linked, so once the adrenals get exhausted, the thyroid also goes low. Pay a visit to your doctor to get them checked if you suspect that your thyroid does not function well enough. Swap your regular toothpaste for a fluoride-free one as studies have shown that fluoride interferes with the thyroid function. The Food and Drug Administration (FDA) has acknowledged potential risks and requires a poison warning on every tube of toothpaste now sold in the USA.

When I first learned about all of the toxic ingredients in my food, personal and household products, I felt quite overwhelmed and unsure where to start. It was also becoming more evident to me that no wonder I had been so increasingly ill if all of these toxins were poisoning my body. Combined, they were perpetuating a severe hormonal imbalance, inflammation and estrogen dominance as well as feeding my endometriosis.

I appreciate that when you first read the above, it might feel like a BIG adjustment to your life. But I promise you it is so worth it. These products are making you ill and keeping you sick. Endometriosis is 'fed' and inflamed every time you apply a product that is an xenoestrogen.

Start by making small adjustments, as you can afford them. Even just gradual, small improvements will benefit your body and help you heal. But strive to eliminate as many as possible over time. It is crucial to increase your awareness of what produce and products go into your body, on your body, and around your body.

As the Tanzanian Proverb says, *"little by little, a little becomes a lot"*.

Chapter 14 -

The Power of Bioidentical Progesterone Cream

* * *

Minds are like parachutes; they only function when they are
open

– Thomas Dewar

I have described in the earlier chapters how the two main sex

hormones – progesterone and estrogen – must maintain an ideal ratio or a woman's body will go into a state of estrogen dominance. Back in the 1970s, there was a common fundamental misunderstanding about the physiological role of estrogen and progesterone throughout a woman's reproductive life cycle. This resulted in a treatment strategy mostly for menopausal women, which was not based upon scientific evidence. Synthetic estrogen was so idealised back then and progesterone was neglected. This led to significant suffering for premenopausal, peri-menopausal, and postmenopausal women with endometriosis. Studies have shown that for many women who suffered from these uncomfortable and often disabling estrogen dominance symptoms, the mistake of supplementing with synthetic estrogen only aggravated their conditions.[33]

I came to the realisation, once I had removed all the xenoestrogens, that a decrease in progesterone and a significant increase in estrogen (estrogen dominance) is the real culprit behind these estrogen dominant symptoms and disorders like endometriosis, adenomyosis, cysts and fibroids. Disturbingly though, the medical establishment had also identified this but used it as a way to make more money. They discovered a way to boost the progesterone deficiency using the synthetic, pharmaceutically produced progesterone called 'Progestin' and 'Progestogen' (you will note how similar the names are to progesterone, which of course creates greater confusion for women). Even though pharmaceutical companies start off using the original natural progesterone, they then chemically alter it, but it's not identical to what we produce naturally in our bodies. The chemically altered version is called 'progestin'. It allows them to patent the tablets or suppositories etc. that they make and then sell them to medical establishments and hospitals to make sizeable profits. It is this chemical alteration though which makes the synthetic progesterone less effective, as it does not act on target tissues in the same way as natural progesterone would. This can cause several unpleasant side effects, with the most common one being an increased risk of breast cancer.[34]

However, many women have learned to use a natural bioidentical progesterone cream alternative to help in the treatment of endometriosis. Natural bioidentical cream used to be routinely prescribed by doctors in the USA and UK in the 1960s, before the pharmaceutical giants exercised their influence. This treatment regime is among the top choices that help reduce symptoms and aid in the treatment of endometriosis. When applied in a high enough dose, this treatment can induce a safe pseudo pregnancy-like condition that helps stop the further development of endometriosis. The main objective of the bioidentical progesterone is to counteract the estrogen dominance. Using bioidentical progesterone cream also reduces the further proliferation of endometriosis implants and also allows any other implants that are present to shrink. There are no known side effects from taking bioidentical progesterone cream, except for sleepiness when taken in high amounts.

Hormone Testing

I would suggest getting a saliva hormone test done, which is more reliable than a blood test. You may ask your doctor, or order the testing kits – which are inexpensive and can be purchased online. Test for estradiol and progesterone to determine a baseline to give yourself a comparison for the future. There are five ways that estrogen dominance can show up; high estrogen to low progesterone (which is the classic definition of the imbalance), high estrogen to normal progesterone, normal estrogen to low progesterone, low estrogen to low progesterone and normal levels of estrogen and progesterone. Whatever the results, if you are experiencing all of the classic estrogen-dominant and endometriosis symptoms, it is because your body is being bombarded by the many estrogen-mimicking chemicals (xenoestrogens) in our environment.

How to Use Natural Bioidentical Progesterone Cream

The proper procedure for using bioidentical progesterone cream is to apply it from day six of your cycle up until day 26, using one ounce of the cream per week, for three weeks, and then stop just before your expected period. After four to six months of use, you should be noticing that your menstrual pains have gradually subsided, because the monthly bleeding from the endometriosis implants is less and the healing of the inflammatory sites begin to occur.

You may be wondering how these bioidentical hormones are made? In the human body, the ovaries, the testicles, and the adrenal glands manufacture a series of hormones known as steroids that are all derived from cholesterol. In the early 1960s, science was able to synthesise all of these molecules, starting either from cholesterol or from plant steroids found in nature.

Bioidentical hormones are derived from a plant oil called diosgenin, which has a very similar chemical structure to cholesterol. Diosgenin is extracted primarily from wild yams and some bean species but is also found in thousands of other plants worldwide. However, the human body cannot convert this compound into steroid hormones. Diosgenin needs to be chemically altered in a laboratory to precisely match the human steroid hormones. The manufactured molecules now exactly match the chemical structure and the effects of hormones that occur naturally in the human body; hence they are called bioidentical.

The Safe Hormone

Bioidentical progesterone contains the identical chemical structure and composition to the actual progesterone hormone produced in a woman's body. As mentioned earlier, bioidentical progesterone should not be confused with synthetic medical progesterone-like chemicals that the pharmaceutical companies produce – called progestins or progestogens – because these are unnatural to a woman's body. These progestins or progestogens bind to the body's progesterone receptors and function like progesterone, but only temporarily. This happens because progestins or progestogens are chemically different from bioidentical progesterone. They also possess inherent side effects that may cause more harm than good to your already worsening endometriosis situation.

When you go to find a bioidentical progesterone cream, make sure you buy the ones with at least 500mg of natural progesterone per ounce. So shop around, do enough research, and buy the best quality bioidentical progesterone cream you can afford for the treatment of your endometriosis condition, or look at my online resources page for recommended products at https://HealEndometriosisNaturally.com/Resources

In the UK, some doctors can often prescribe a progesterone cream if they are fundholding practices, or if the Area Health Authority will pay. Be careful when using bioidentical pills or suppositories as the body tends to break down the progesterone supplied through these methods before it can reach receptors.

Upon application, rub the cream on the parts of your body that have good circulation such as the breasts, neck, legs, chest, arms, thighs, soles of the feet, and the back. If you have a lot of body fat, the progesterone will be soaked up by that body fat first, before being absorbed into your bloodstream. This means you will have to apply a higher dose to make it effective.

What should you do if you start to feel an increase in estrogen dominance symptoms after applying bioidentical progesterone cream?

Experts would say that the introduction of progesterone may temporarily stimulate the body's estrogen dormant receptor sites. As we all know, progesterone is the direct counterpart of estrogen, and it is normal for estrogen to react when progesterone is first introduced.

Suppose your bioidentical progesterone cream seems to have no effect on your condition. In that case, the most obvious answer to this is an inferior quality product, or the dosage needs to be increased.

If you have been using your bioidentical progesterone cream for more than 60-90 days as recommended by most manufacturers and you do not see any improvement in your symptoms, then this is unusual. Therefore you should consider changing your brand as it may not be a high enough dosage or good enough quality. Also, ensure to have another look around your personal and household products to see what xenoestrogens or phytoestrogens might still be lurking around and affecting or adding inflammation to your body.

So I had made a conscious effort to remove all known toxins from my personal and household products, and the application of natural bioidentical progesterone cream made a tremendous difference to my body, and still does today.

Combined with a few other factors, which I will be explaining in later chapters, natural bioidentical progesterone cream helped with the reduction of many of my endometriosis symptoms including: breast pain, stomach cramps, reduction in blood flow, and premenstrual syndrome.

And the best part of it all: it was all-natural, compatible with my body, and there were no side effects!

Finally, I was back in the driving seat of my body.

Chapter 15 -

The Endometriosis Power Protein Shake

* * *

The only thing you have to fear is fear itself
— Franklin D Roosevelt

I t is usual for women with endometriosis to look at protein

shakes and get the impression that these nutritious drinks are only for men or bodybuilders. However, this is not quite true. A woman's body does not produce enough testosterone to build muscle in the same way as a man's body. Yet, this does not mean women cannot benefit from eating a diet adequate in protein. High-protein shakes, and indeed all high-protein foods, help develop lean muscle mass by supplying the body with the necessary amino acids for building and repairing tissue. These effects can be of benefit for women. It is also true that these shakes increase satiety, deliver essential nutrients, improve energy and metabolic activity. Also, they tend to be lower in calories (which can help people lose fat) and due to their powdered format they are very easy to digest.

Protein is known as the building block nutrient of our bodies as it supplies us with all 20 amino acids; nine of which are vital for survival. Amino acids are critical in maintaining our body tissue, including the development and repair of our hair, our skin, our eyes, and our muscles and organs – which are all made from proteins. This is the main reason why children and athletes need more protein per pound of bodyweight than the average adult. They are growing and developing new tissue.

Let us get a better understanding of the role of protein in our body. Protein is a fundamental substance found in every cell in the human body. Other than water, protein is the most abundant substance in our body. It is a critical component in every cell as it is what makes up our enzymes, antibodies, and helps with messages, transport, and storage throughout the body.

These proteins are synthesised by ribosomes – small proteins themselves that transcribe our DNA (transferred by messenger RNA) and form polypeptide chains, utilising the amino acids from the dietary protein we consume. These polypeptide chains then go on to develop complex chains (secondary, tertiary, and quaternary structures) with one another through hydrogen bonds and further peptide bonds. These complex chains are called proteins. As protein is used in many vital processes in our bodies, it needs to be consistently replaced. We can accomplish this by regularly consuming foods that are rich in high-quality protein.

Protein's primary function is in repairing and regenerating cells, but just like fats and carbohydrates it can also be a source of energy for our body. If we consume more protein than we need for body tissue maintenance and other functions, our body will use it for energy.

Interestingly protein is very much involved in creating hormones. Proteins help control body functions that involve the interaction of several organs. For example, insulin (a small protein) helps regulate blood sugar which interacts with organs such as the pancreas and the liver. Another example of a protein hormone, secretin assists in the digestive process by stimulating the pancreas and the intestines to create the necessary digestive juices.

Protein is a major facilitator in transporting specific molecules inside our body. Haemoglobin, for example, is a globular protein with an iron ion in it that transports oxygen throughout our body. Apart from transportation, protein also acts as storage for specific molecules. Another example is ferritin, which combines with iron for storage in the liver.

Another significant role that protein plays in our body is in the formation of antibodies. Antibodies help prevent infection, illness, and disease. These proteins are the ones that identify and assist in destroying antigens, such as bacteria and viruses. These proteins, released by a type of white blood cell called a B lymphocyte, often work in conjunction with the other white blood cells like macrophages and neutrophils. There are many types of antibodies, and consequently multiple ways in which they work, but here are the most common:

- Neutralisation – Antibodies bind to the surface of a pathogen and neutralise/inhibit its negative biological effect on the body.

- Agglutination – Antibodies attach themselves to pathogens and then clump them together so that it is easier for phagocytes to find, engulf and digest the pathogens via phagocytosis.

- Fixation – In which antibodies bind to the surface of pathogens and cause them to lyse (explode), thus killing them and neutralising their threat.

Boost your body

The problem with a lot of women with endometriosis is that they are in such chronic pain that they lose their appetites and do not feel like eating. I often used to go through the whole day without having breakfast or lunch, and wonder why later in the afternoon I felt ill and tired. I would graze on sugar and chocolate to get energy hits (which releases dopamine; a feel-good feeling in the brain) to help me get through the rest of the day.

Now we know how important it is to maintain enough proteins in our body. If for some reason, you cannot get enough protein from solid food, protein shakes are your best alternative to tackle your protein deficiency.

There are so many different kinds of protein shakes sold in the market, but it is essential that you should look out for the organic ones that are free from additives and bulking agents. Make sure to avoid ones that contain whey or soy protein and sugar or sweeteners. Ideally, consume organic rice or pea protein powder.

Replacing your meals with protein shakes whilst you recover can help you consume the calories and nutrients your body needs to repair and heal. It can also give you the energy your body requires to function in a day. You will eventually want to start eating solid food again once the pain reduces, but in the meantime, you may find it easier to 'drink' your food.

At the beginning, aim to have at least one protein shake every day, but try to progress to having two or even three a day. It is important to have your shake at breakfast as it will set you up for the day. To make it, I recommend a one-litre glass of still mineral or filtered water or coconut milk, with one serving scoop (two tablespoons) of rice or pea organic protein powder, two crushed best quality multivitamin and mineral tablets (or use a rice-based multivitamin and mineral powder) and then top it up with nutritious green powder, like chlorella or spirulina that must be wheat-free and free from added sugar/sweetener.

As you are recovering, I encourage you to integrate these protein shakes into your diet because of the numerous benefits they can give you. Always make sure that there is no wheat or added sugar in the ingredients. Whenever possible, it is still best to make your protein shakes from fresh ingredients. This will keep you away from the synthetic ingredients that are included in off-the-shelf protein shakes sold in the supermarkets.

When you do start to eat solid proteins again, please ensure they are good quality, hormone-free, grass-fed, and free-range meat and poultry. Protein has had a lot of bad press over the years, and alternatives like 'Quorn' and tofu have sprung up, but they are inferior alternatives to animal protein, fish, pulses, beans, nuts, and seeds.

I had been completely ignorant about the vital role of protein in the healing of our bodies. I have now realised that the only food sources our cavemen and women ancestors would have lived off for thousands of years would have been protein, nuts, seeds and fruit.

Our Western society has expanded so rapidly over the past 80 years that governments have had to adjust to feeding the population quickly and readily – hence the growth in the use of versatile, easy-to-produce crops like wheat, corn and soy.

I suddenly saw food in a whole new light, and it did not seem so complicated after all. And the best part was there were no nasty side effects.

It was bye-bye the bakers and hello nature.

Chapter 16 -

The Use of Multivitamin and Mineral Supplements

* * *

You gain strength, courage and confidence by every experience in which you really stop to look fear in the face
— *Eleanor Roosevelt*

There may be instances where you cannot get full access to

all the best sources of nutrients through a well-balanced diet of protein power shakes or solid food. In this case, your other option is to slowly introduce vitamins and mineral supplements to augment your daily healthy eating habits.

We are what we eat, but why does what we eat these days lack the nutrition content we so badly need? Many of the foods we consume in the Western world have travelled great distances and are not grown locally. The issue here is that to travel great distances, those foods are likely picked early and are sprayed with chemical pesticides to slow down the ripening process. As such, these chemicals can create issues for our health, and produce that has been picked too early may lack the nutrients that we need.

Many women with endometriosis have nutritional deficiencies and require supplementation for a short to medium period. Iron deficiencies are common for those with a history of prolonged blood loss over many years. Ask your doctor to check your ferritin iron levels, and even if they come back within range but are on the low side, consider taking a non-constipating iron supplement every day for 3 months. This will work wonders for your body and has been shown to improve things such as hair thickness and energy levels.

To replenish your body's nutrients – which can help it to recover more quickly – take a good quality (without things like talc, bulking agents, wheat or sugar/sweeteners) multivitamin and mineral tablet or powder every day. Please get the best quality you can afford as the cheap versions are filled with nasty bulking agents. Other supplements worth considering on top of a multivitamin are as follows.

Magnesium

Magnesium is a mineral that is present in relatively large amounts in our body. Estimates show that an average person's body contains 25 grams of magnesium, half of which is in the bones. Magnesium is vital in more than 300 biochemical reactions that keep our body working. It is required for the proper growth and maintenance of our bones. It is also responsible for the proper function of our nerves, muscles, and many other parts of our bodies. In the stomach, for example, it helps to neutralise stomach acid and to move stools conveniently through the intestine.

A sign you may be deficient in magnesium is a constant craving for chocolate. Chocolate has high levels of magnesium in it, which is why some people desire it. Restless, itchy, and unsettled sensations in the legs, especially at night, can be an indication of magnesium deficiency too, and also of estrogen dominance. Other signs can include, but are not limited to: fatigue, high blood pressure, an irregular heartbeat, and muscle weakness.

Zinc

Zinc is a metal and called an 'essential trace element' because only tiny amounts of it are necessary for human health. It is essential for enzyme activity, helping cells to reproduce, thereby assisting our bodies regenerate and repair. Zinc also plays a vital role in our immune system. Moreover, zinc is present in high concentrations in our eyes and is involved in maintaining good vision. Zinc is a catalyst for 100 enzymes in the body. Other roles include protein synthesis, wound healing and the maintenance of proper taste and smell. Common signs that show your body is low in zinc include slowed growth, loss of appetite, low insulin levels, irritability, generalised hair loss, slow wound healing, rough and dry skin, reduced sense of taste and smell, diarrhoea, and nausea. Zinc picolinate is best for absorption. A daily intake of zinc is required as the body has no specialised way of storing it.

Calcium

When our menstrual period draws near, the calcium level in our body decreases. This creates a calcium deficiency which can lead to symptoms such as muscle cramps, headaches, osteoporosis, and pelvic pain. Calcium is a mineral that is a vital part of our bones and teeth. Our heart, nerves, and blood-clotting systems require calcium to work properly. Calcium helps to relieve premenstrual syndrome, leg cramps, high blood pressure, and reduces the risk of colon and rectal cancers. Our bones and teeth contain over 99% of the calcium present in our body. The rest is found in the blood, muscles, and other tissues. It serves functions in those other tissues such as mediating vasoconstriction and vasodilation, muscle contraction, nerve transmission, and glandular secretion – to name a few. Calcium in our bones acts as a reserve and is released in the body when it is needed. This process occurs mostly in women during pregnancy, as the unborn infant is also supplied with calcium in the womb. As we age, the calcium concentration in our body declines because it is released through sweat, skin cells, and waste. Our bones are constantly breaking down and rebuilding, so we need to take extra calcium supplements to help to stay strong. Calcium D-glucarate is best, as it has been shown to help with detoxification in the body and decreases the toxicity of xenoestrogens in the bowel as it promotes excretion.

Iron

Iron is a mineral and most of it is found in the haemoglobin of red blood cells and the myoglobin of skeletal muscle cells. As iron is a vital part of haemoglobin, it is therefore responsible for transporting oxygen and carbon dioxide. In red blood cells, iron is part of the central heme group, which is surrounded by four haemoglobin subunits. Each subunit can carry one molecule of oxygen but for them to be able to do this the central heme group must have bound to an oxygen molecule first. The only way this can happen though is if there is an iron ion in the heme group. Therefore, if red blood cells do not have enough iron available, then their haemoglobin will be unable to bind to any oxygen, and our cells will become deprived of this essential gas – and thus we see the importance of iron in the body. Women with endometriosis who suffer from very heavy periods and excessive blood loss can develop an iron deficiency, causing them to become anaemic. This can mainly be characterised by grey pallor, extreme fatigue, and weakness.

Selenium

Selenium is a mineral, and most of it in our body comes from our diet. The amount of selenium consumed depends on where we live in the world. Examples of good selenium sources are crabs, liver, fish, and poultry. The amount of selenium available varies widely, meaning that fish found in Europe will contain different levels of selenium from fish found in Asia, even though they might be the same species of fish. Selenium is used against diseases relating to the heart and blood vessels, including a stroke and the 'hardening of the arteries'. Selenium also seems to increase the action of antioxidants. Researchers have reported that selenium, when taken together with vitamins E and C, was associated with a decrease in the severity of the endometriosis condition.[35]

B Vitamins

These vitamins are essential for the breakdown of proteins, carbohydrates, and fats in our body. They are responsible for energy metabolism, for a standard functioning nervous system, and for the reduction of tiredness and fatigue. One very important B vitamin is folic acid. All of the doctors in the world recommend that any woman of childbearing age must take a folic acid supplement. The main reason is folic acid can protect against congenital disabilities that may form before a woman knows she is pregnant.

Another important B vitamin is vitamin B12, otherwise known as cobalamin. Vitamin B12 plays a role in DNA synthesis and maintenance and helps keep our nerve cells and red blood cells healthy. Vitamin B3, or non-flush niacinamide, is another B vitamin that is good for your body. It is vital to have large quantities of niacinamide in our bodies, to remain in good health. When used as a treatment, higher amounts of B3 can improve cholesterol levels and lower the risks of cardiovascular complications. B7 is particularly useful for reversing hair loss and thickening hair. B vitamins are also water-soluble, so any excess that gets consumed will be flushed out of the body through urination and sweating.

Vitamin C

Vitamin C, or ascorbic acid, is the most well-known immune system booster and is involved in almost all types of tissue repair as well as being great for wound healing. Most experts still recommend getting vitamin C from a diet rich in fruits and vegetables, for example, freshly-squeezed orange juice. I also recommend supplementing with vitamin C capsules sometimes when you are run down or injured. Our body also uses vitamin C to build and maintain collagen. Since vitamin C is a water-soluble vitamin, the body can extract its requirements and flush out any excess through urine or sweat.

Vitamin A

This is another well-known supplement for boosting our immune systems. This vitamin is easily found in many fruits, vegetables, eggs, whole milk, butter, meat, and oily saltwater fish. Vitamin A helps women who experience heavy menstrual periods, premenstrual syndrome, vaginal infections, 'lumpy' breasts, and breast cancer. Pregnant and breast-feeding women who are diagnosed with HIV take vitamin A to decrease the risk of transmitting HIV to the baby.

Vitamin E

The main benefit of vitamin E is in its capacity as an antioxidant. This means that it helps to slow down the processes that age and damage our cells. Vitamin E helps the distribution and oxygen-carrying capacities of our haemoglobin. This is one of the reasons why we see women who look 30 even when they are, in fact, 50 years old. They have sufficient concentrations of vitamin E within their system. Vitamin E is also used to lessen the harmful effects of medical treatments, such as dialysis and radiation. People who take medication for hair loss and lung damage consume vitamin E to reduce unwanted side effects. Taking vitamin E can help to prevent premenstrual syndrome, excruciating periods, menopausal syndrome, hot flashes, breast cysts and complications in late pregnancy due to high blood pressure.

Fish Oil

The reason fish oils are so good for the body is that they are almost entirely composed of omega-3 fatty acids. Omega-3 fatty acids are essential for our bodies, and taking sufficient amounts can help to reduce inflammation, improve skin tone and strengthen joints. In the Western world, most people are very deficient in omega-3. You may be wondering why I am not suggesting supplementing with omega-6-9 fatty acids. Well, the Western diet is already very abundant in those two omegas, but it severely lacks omega-3. So, supplement with omega-3 fatty acids and, because not every fish oil is made the same, please get the best your money can buy.

Probiotics

The widespread use of antibiotics in the Western world alongside factors like drinking, smoking, overeating sugar, and a lack of exercise means that the amount of healthy intestinal gut flora in our bodies has diminished. Replenishing the 'good' bacteria is essential for fighting off invading pathogens and promoting the repair of damaged tissue, so supplement with Lactobacillus acidophilus, preferably containing Bifidobacteria.

So there you have it, a list of essential multivitamins and minerals that I use and that will support your body into a recovery and repair state. Most of the vitamins and supplements I have described here can be bought easily online. It is crucial, as I stated earlier, that you make sure you purchase good quality vitamins, ensuring they are not full of sugar or fillers like chalk, talc, or soy.

Consult with your doctor, chemist, or pharmacist if you are concerned in any way prior to taking any supplements, especially if you are concerned that they might interfere with any current medications.

Ideally, it would be best to have a doctor to support you in your desire to address your endometriosis naturally. Ask him or her to work with you, and indeed use you as a case study to help other women. If complications arise in any way, shape, or form, contact your doctor who can readily make changes. They can take a look at why you are experiencing a reaction.

Always start slowly with any supplement – introducing only one supplement at a time. This is important; your body has been through enough stress, especially women who have had surgery, which is a traumatic experience on the body. All women with endometriosis have had to endure prolonged, intense periods of pain and upset, and this can make your body incredibly sensitive to ingredients. Introduce supplements slowly to gauge your bodies response to them and ensure sure that you do not have any undiscovered allergies to these supplements.

If you find a supplement is too potent in its capsule dose form, then open the capsule and split the dose up. I was so ill when I started taking tablets that I had to split many of the supplements into four doses and then slowly increase the dosage as my body adjusted. Remember the aim is to get you well, not to make you worse, so go slow. Slow is fast!.

Chapter 17 -

Natural Aromatase Inhibitors

* * *

*If you always do, what you have always done, you will always
get, what you've always gotten*

— Wendy K Laidlaw

I f you find you have removed all environmental toxins, changed

over your personal products (including creams, lotions and perfumes), swapped your household products, are drinking protein shakes, eating hormone-free meats and avoiding wheat, sugar and soy, supplementing with multivitamins and minerals, as well as supplementing with natural bioidentical progesterone cream and are still experiencing pain, then it may be time to look at another layer in the battle against estrogen dominance and endometriosis in the body.

As we have discussed, estrogen dominance is a hormonal imbalance of excess estrogen and low levels of progesterone caused by a combination of poor diet, nutritional deficiencies, xenoestrogens, dioxins, and phytoestrogens. These factors cause estrogen levels to increase in the body and inhibit the liver's ability to breakdown and expel estrogen. If you are poorly nourished from your diet and have high estrogen, chances are you may have high levels of the enzyme aromatase. Excess aromatase in the body means that the inflammation cycle of endometriosis will be perpetuated.

Excess estrogen can also affect both the adrenal and thyroid glands, which in turn can make estrogen dominance worse. This is where natural aromatase inhibitors might be considered as an additional way of supporting your body into balance.

What is Aromatase?

Aromatase or estrogen synthase is an enzyme involved in the production of estrogen. It does this by increasing the conversion of androgens (hormones such as testosterone) to one of the three estrogens called estradiol and estrone. Aromatase is located in estrogen-producing cells in the ovaries, adrenal glands, testicles, fat tissue, and the brain.

Natural aromatase inhibitors prevent the aromatase enzyme, and in doing so, lowers the level of two of the estrogens: estradiol and estrone. You will not be surprised to hear that medical aromatase inhibitors, prescribed by doctors and consultants, have side effects. Natural aromatase inhibitors are available in supplement form, although one natural way to acquire aromatase is to eat vegetables rich in indole-3-carbinole.

In addition to increasing my intake of organic kale, cauliflower, and broccoli, I've listed below some of the natural aromatase inhibitor supplements I used in my natural journey

I3C

I3C stands for 'indole-3 carbinole', which is found naturally in vegetables like cabbage, cauliflower, and broccoli. I3C is a precursor to diindolylmethane (DIM). I3C is available in supplement form.

Diindolylmethane (DIM)

DIM is a compound derived from the digestion of indole-3-carbinole, found in cruciferous vegetables such as broccoli, brussels sprouts, cabbage, and kale. It is also available in supplement form. DIM is purported to produce changes in the metabolism of unhealthy excess estrogen-like estradiol, whilst increasing levels of healthy estrogens like estriol.

Myomin

Myomin is a formula of Chinese herbs produced by Chi's Enterprise and contains natural ingredients Aralia, Smilax glabra, Curcuma zedoria, and Cyperus rotundus. These herbs have traditionally been used for various female ailments and hormone-related disorders. Clinical trials show that myomin helps metabolise unhealthy estrogens (estradiol and estrone) into the good form of estrogen (estriol). Myomin is a natural aromatase inhibitor and helps support over-worked adrenal glands. Curcuma has also been found to have antioxidant, antiviral, anti-inflammatory, and immune-boosting effects.

Calcium D-glucarate

If I3C, DIM and myomin do not help you get the desired results, you may want first to consider increasing the dosage, and then adding calcium D-glucarate to your regimen. Calcium D-glucarate helps to make sure that hormones are not reabsorbed into the bloodstream (from where they may be deposited in the cells and tissue), but expelled from the body.

It has also been suggested that zinc and vitamin E can also act as aromatase inhibitors.

The natural aromatase inhibitors were particularly helpful in the elimination of all of my adenomyosis symptoms. Encouragingly for me, within a few weeks of taking the tablets, the dragging sensations, contractions, 'bearing down' heaviness and vaginal pain had disappeared.

Despite being told by the gynaecologist that the only solution was to have my uterus cut out, I had successfully identified the sources of my troubles, and I had proved the doctors wrong again.

Chapter 18 -

Systemic Enzyme Therapy

* * *

Twenty years from now, you will be more disappointed at the
things you didn't do, than by the ones you did
— Mark Twain

E nzymes are biological molecules (typically proteins) that

are required for every single chemical action that takes place in your body. To put it simply, they work by speeding up biological reactions. All of your cells and systems depend upon enzymes – from your organs, muscles, bones, and tissues to your immune system, digestive system, bloodstream, spleen, liver, kidneys, and pancreas. This also influences your ability to see, think, feel, and breathe.

In the immune system, macrophages (the Greek name for "big eaters"), which are a type of phagocyte, produce a wide array of powerful chemical substances including cytokines and enzymes. These enzymes are secreted in response to infection, and dead or damaged cells. The job of the macrophage enzymes is to remove any cellular debris or dead cells that are found where they should not be.

Macrophages, because they are phagocytes, also get rid of pathogens by engulfing and then digesting them with digestive enzymes. As we already know, the displacement of endometrial tissue in the abdomen, endometrial lesions, cysts, and adhesions are what macrophages are designed to 'clean up'. However, in women with endometriosis, they do not do their job well.

Serrapeptase

Systemic Enzyme Therapy has a long history of being used in Germany, central Europe, Japan, and Mexico since the 1950s, and is still used there today. One enzyme called serrapeptase is used frequently in this therapy. It is a proteolytic enzyme found in the intestines of silkworms and is used to digest the protective cocoon of the silkworm, enabling it to emerge and fly away. It is now created through a natural fermentation process in laboratories. What is unique about this enzyme is that it can dissolve non-living tissue but does not in any way damage living cells. Its main benefits include digesting dead cells or unwanted tissue and having analgesic, anti-oedema, fibrinolytic and anti-inflammatory properties. Its positive effects have been widely documented in several clinical studies and reviews. For example, it was used during a double-blind study by German researchers on 66 patients. They discovered that those receiving serrapeptase had a 50% reduction in swelling within three days of surgery compared to the two control groups which had no such reduction. Also, there was a much faster decrease in the pain of the serrapeptase-taking patients than the patients in the control groups, and within ten days, they had no pain.[36] As you can see, you will assist your body in 'eating up' adhesions, cysts, and endometrial debris through systemic enzyme therapy supplementation and by consuming serrapeptase.

Systemic enzyme formulas are used to treat joint inflammation, pain, inflammation, blood clots, Alzheimer's, angina, multiple sclerosis, prostatitis, and respiratory infections. Serrapeptase helps to naturally dissolve the billions of dead cells in the body, without harming any living tissue.

Many times I visited and asked doctors and gynaecologists why this product was not used or prescribed in the UK. Serrapeptase is used routinely in other countries as it is so safe, so effective and importantly has no side effects – and it is an excellent alternative to painkillers. Its effectiveness has been validated in over 40 clinical trials, and it has been used for over 30 years by many millions of people in Asia and Europe.

With regards to the quantity of serrapeptase to take, I started with capsules of 80,000 IU. I moved up to 250,000 IU once I felt confident my body was happy with them. However, as I always caution, and even though there are no known side effects and it is ordinarily well-tolerated, please do start with smaller doses first to check how your body responds to them. After a few days, you should begin to increase it slowly until you feel the positive effects.

Nattokinase

Nattokinase is another natural enzyme supplement that speeds up the biochemical reactions in the body. Like serrapeptase, nattokinase has been scientifically proven to benefit the cardiovascular system, reduce blood clots and varicose veins, and to improve the circulatory systems. Nattokinase works by breaking down 'fibrins' which are the fibres of blood clots and adhesions, and they then dispel them from the body. Recent studies of this powerful enzyme have shown its effectiveness in reducing fibroids and cysts in women. Nattokinase is extracted from nattō – boiled soybeans that have been fermented with a bacterium called Bacillus natto. I was apprehensive about trying this supplement when I heard that it was made from soybeans. I contacted a few suppliers directly, and I was reassured many times that although it is made from soybeans, the process of making nattokinase takes the estrogenic compounds out it.

Digestive Enzymes

Our body produces digestive enzymes that are primarily created in the pancreas and small intestine. These enzymes help our body breakdown food so it can be absorbed in the intestines. When your body has been on pain killers, drugs, and had surgery over prolonged periods of time, or been under extended periods of stress which inhibit natural enzyme production, the digestive process needs to be restored to a healthy balance. You will know if you need to supplement with digestive enzymes if you have any of the following symptoms:

- Undigested food in your stool
- Bloating after meals, gas, or flatulence
- Hard sensation in your stomach
- Chronic fatigue
- Sugar cravings
- Fatigue or sleep issues
- Skin inflammation and acne

Unfortunately, our cooked or processed foods destroy any enzymes that were naturally in the food, so you can see again why it is essential to eat raw and freshly made food, or supplement if required.

Systemic enzyme therapy was the final piece of my endometriosis body puzzle. It took a few weeks to introduce the tablets, and I slowly built them up to the point where I was taking serrapeptase, nattokinase, and digestive enzymes two to three times a day.

In addition to a continued reduction in pain, I also noticed positive changes in other areas of my body. This included the regularity of my bowel movements (I had always suffered from terrible constipation), my nails got thicker, and the small surface cysts (on my ankle and my nose) disappeared.

Finally, as with all other supplements, make sure that you read the ingredients list thoroughly. You would be surprised what some unscrupulous manufacturers pop into their capsules. You get what you pay for, so go for the best you can afford. I recommend capsules over tablets as they are easier to digest. How long you need to supplement for will depend on each person but for me it was three months.

Chapter 19 -

Herbal Medicine

* * *

In the middle of difficulty lies opportunity
                                    – Albert Einstein

L et us begin to discuss herbal medicines. Herbal medicines
are usually prepared by using the roots, flowers, stems, leaves, or barks
of plants with medicinal properties. These preparations can be inhaled,
applied as a topical salve, inserted as a suppository, or ingested orally
in a tablet form or as a drink (like tea). Often, different kinds of herbs
are combined to increase the effects.

One beneficial effect from herbal medicine for endometriosis
sufferers is the impact it can have on reducing excess levels of estrogen
in the body. We already know that the liver is the main organ that
breaks down estrogen, and herbalists suggest that the herbal medicine
to be prepared should target the welfare and health of the liver. The
most notable herbal preparation that is known to stimulate liver
function is the combination of dandelion, beet leaves, Cascara sagrada
and Arctostaphylos uva ursi. The effect is not immediate. However,

give it a few months of regular intake, and one will feel free of symptomatic pain.

Various other herbs and plant foods that help relieve endometriosis and symptomatic pain include: cranberry, plantain, blue cohosh, St. John's wort, peppermint, valerian, false unicorn, dong quai, evening primrose oil, chasteberry, black cohosh, uva ursi, couchgrass, red raspberry, yam, and white willow.

Chinese Herbs

In China, the treatment of endometriosis through the use of Chinese Herbal Medicine (CHM) is routine. There has been considerable research conducted into the role of CHM and its role in alleviating pain, promoting fertility, and preventing relapse. Some studies claim that oral CHM may provide better overall treatment for relieving painful menstruation and shrinking cysts or lumps when used in conjunction with a Chinese Herbal Medicine enema.

Keishi-bukuryo-gan (KBG) is a traditional Chinese herbal remedy and has been an approved prescription medication since the 1970s. Keishi-bukuryo-gan has been used for the treatment of gynaecological disorders, such as hypermenorrhea, dysmenorrhea, and infertility. It is also very popular in Japan, where some 40 million prescriptions are handed out each year.

Shakuyaku-kanzo-tos (SKT) is a herbal formula traditionally used in Japan, Korea, and China. Studies have shown it reduces cysts, and it is known to relieve menstrual pain, muscle spasm, and muscle pain.

Other helpful herbs

Vitex agnus-castus is popular in Europe for relieving menstrual difficulties and increasing natural progesterone production.

Chrysin is a naturally occurring flavonoid in chamomile, passion flowers, honeycombs, and certain mushrooms. It is a natural estrogen aromatase blocker, stopping testosterone from converting into estrogen.

Cramp bark is a natural herb that helps to ease uterine cramps during menstruation.

French maritime pine bark (also known as pycnogenol) is a powerful antioxidant which can also help to metabolise excess estrogen and restore hair loss.

Milk Thistle (Silybum marianum) is a wonderful herb that can help with liver detoxification. If I ever indulge in a glass of alcohol, I take two tablets before drinking and then I take two more before I go to bed with a glass of water.

Asparagus extract is a useful herb for helping your kidneys detoxify.

As with all medications, drugs, supplements, or herbs, please do your own research before consuming them and consult your doctor if you have any reactions.

Chapter 20 -

Endometriosis Alternatives and Other Complementary Therapy

* * *

The quality of a person's life is in direct proportion to their commitment to excellence, regardless of their chosen field of endeavour

— Vince Lombardi

O ver the years, millions of women suffering from

endometriosis have sought relief for their symptoms. Tired and fed up with the conventional medical approach, some of them tried to follow the complementary therapy way. These therapies may include any healing method from the use of herbs to various pain management techniques. Many suffering women can adopt them in an attempt to alleviate, or otherwise manage a number of symptoms, non-invasively.

Acupuncture

This ancient and traditional Chinese medicine involves fine needles inserted at specific sites in the body for therapeutic or preventive purposes. This is based on the belief that an energy, or life force, flows through our bodies via channels called meridians. Practitioners of acupuncture who adhere to this belief believe that when this life force does not flow freely through our body, this will cause illness. The insertion of the fine needles is considered to restore the flow of this life force and thus restore health.

Acupuncture has been around for centuries and is still being applied today to treat pain conditions such as headaches, lower back pains, and osteoarthritis. It has also been reported to help people with conditions ranging from infertility to anxiety and asthma. There are also some reports that acupuncture works for other problems, such as neck pain and post-chemotherapy nausea and vomiting.

Acupuncture relieves general pain and is said to bring relief to women suffering from endometriosis pain, menstrual cramping, and even post-operative pain. Unfortunately, acupuncture is not readily available worldwide. There are even countries that have outlawed it.

Myofascial Massage

Myofascial release massage is a specialised physical treatment for releasing tensions and restrictions caused by adhesions in the pelvic area. 'Myo' means muscle and 'fascia' means band. Fascia is connective tissue made of elastin and collagen fibres, surrounded by a viscous fluid. These two fibre types allow it to be very tough, yet have a high degree of flexibility, and it can respond well to manipulation through abdominal massage. Women with endometriosis can suffer from many adhesions that form due to inflammation or after surgery. Myofascial massage is an excellent natural alternative to having another operation to remove adhesions that may be wrapped around your internal organs. Another surgery may cause more adhesions, and so the endless cycle would continue.

Myofascial massage was terrific in helping break down my abdominal adhesions. The massage focuses on the abdomen area and is a very safe and effective technique, which releases the tightness of any fixed or tight adhesions into moveable and elastic fibres.

After my 6th surgery, I was in terrible pain and had tightness in my abdomen. The myofascial masseuse was aghast when I turned up at her door, as I was hunched over, looking like an 90-year-old woman, shuffling my feet and unable to stand up straight.

The treatment involves the therapist lifting and turning the abdominal skin and manipulating the layers underneath. It sounds painful, but it was merely a little uncomfortable at times. The treatment was worth the minimal discomfort as within a few weeks I was able to stand up straighter and have less pelvic pain. It took about 12 massage sessions before I started to feel more flexibility and fluidity in my abdomen.

TENS Electrotherapy

Transcutaneous Electrical Nerve Stimulation, or TENS, is the most commonly used electrical stimulation device to apply electrotherapy to the body for the treatment of pain. It has electrodes that can be placed over the area of pain or the nerve supplying the area of pain. The user then can adjust the desired intensity of electrical stimulation and select a high or low frequency. The exact mechanism of electrical stimulation's beneficial effects is not known. However, it is thought that TENS may effectively treat pain by blocking the transmission of pain signals along the nerves. It also shows that electrical stimulation promotes the release of endorphin hormones, which are natural painkillers produced by our bodies.

Shiatsu

Shiatsu, which is also known as acupressure, is a Japanese finger-pressure technique that is similar to massage. With the same purpose as acupuncture, shiatsu is designed to help regulate the flow of energy within the body. This type of massage helps produce deep relaxation and increased energy levels. Apart from relaxation, shiatsu also has other benefits, such as: preventing skin wrinkling, relieving rheumatoid arthritis and muscle pain, relieving migraine headaches, easing women from menstrual cramps, aiding women in labour, helping babies turn in the womb, and improving the circulatory and digestive systems.

Thought Field Therapy (TFT) and Emotional Freedom Technique (EFT)

Thought Field Therapy was created by the psychotherapist Dr Robert Callaghan when a patient of his had a water phobia which after many years could not be cured. Quite by accident, after reading about the meridian systems used in acupuncture, Dr Callaghan discovered that if you 'tapped' on the acupuncture point with your fingers, then stagnant energy would move, and along with it the negative thoughts or anxious feelings.

I have to admit to being a little cynical and resistant to the idea of TFT and EFT when I first heard about them. However, I admit now that I am a complete convert. It is a straightforward process but very effective. There are lots of videos on YouTube showing you how to do it – why not give it a try?

Exercise

Exercise can be a stress reliever and is also a good depression fighter. This is because it improves people's moods by stimulating various brain chemicals that will leave people feeling happier and more relaxed. However, exercise for many women with endometriosis is a point of controversy. It is hard to exercise when your body is wracked with pain, bloating and tenderness. Many women feel guilty or push through the pain and exercise anyway.

Usually, in the beginning, I recommend all gentle types of exercise like walking, swimming, Pilates, or yoga, rather than running, calisthenics or weightlifting. I really enjoy yoga and Pilates, which are relatively delicate forms of exercise that work at strengthening, lengthening and relaxing muscles without causing too much stress on your already tender body. Even going to sit outside in the garden or in a park for 20 minutes a day has beneficial effects for the body and mind. Also, sitting out when it is sunny helps to improve your vitamin D levels naturally.

You can maybe explore more strenuous forms of exercise when you are better, more energised, and your body has healed. The most important thing to remember is to go slowly and gently.

After all, endometriosis is a workout on its own.

Stress Management

Continual chronic levels of unremitting stress in the work place or in a toxic relationship can add a lot of pressure to your already pained body, so whenever possible make time for yourself to rest and relax. You can do this through relaxation exercises, breathing exercises, or mindful meditation (as mentioned earlier). This might be a challenge to start with but over time it will become a habit.

When stress management was first suggested to me, I became aware of just how difficult it was for me to 'destress' or relax – I was always of the mindset that I was somehow lazy, or that there were loads of things needing to be done. However, eventually I got used to it and now I find myself doing these techniques every day.

Even when I was so ill that I could barely sit up or walk, I knew I had to take decisive steps to get my body into a relaxed and healing state. This was hard work for me initially, but persistence and consistency paid off. After a while, and making an effort to allocate time to restorative rest, I started to notice a difference in my body. I was being less reactive to everyday stressors and being more present in the moment.

Stress can come from many sources – poor diet, xenoestrogens, work pressure and deadlines, emotional mistreatment in relationships, financial insecurity, and (in the case of endometriosis) prolonged pain and lack of information. Other stress factors might include not having a safe environment or living with an aggressive or abusive partner or workmate.

When your body is in a constant state of stress, your nervous system can get stuck in the 'flight or fight' mode – sometimes referred to as a maladaptive state. The 'flight or fight' response is essential when you are faced with a sabre-toothed tiger and is designed to protect you from danger. However, as mentioned earlier, to remain in this highly vigilant state for long periods can add more stress and perpetuate any problems in your body. For example, the digestive tract stops functioning. Food consumed may not be broken down properly, causing irritation and inflammation and conditions like irritable bowel syndrome (IBS).

Turn off your mobile phone, unplug your house phone, and create a sign for your bedroom door saying, 'Relaxation in Progress:

DO NOT DISTURB'. Take some essential 'Me Time'. That was what I had to do for myself to carve out the necessary escape from people and situations that were demanding my attention.

I was so good at being there for other people, but could barely look after myself. You need to dedicate time to yourself because you are worth it (just as the L'Oréal advert says).

Your body requires regular rest so it can have a chance to repair and recover. I suggest that a minimum of 20 minutes a day (or more) be allocated to trying some or all of the techniques. I hope you find the above suggestions to be as restorative as I do.

Chapter 21 -

The Basic Principles

* * *

*The difference between the impossible and the possible lies
within the person's determination*

— Tommy Lasorda

L ike any new routine, at the start it may be challenging. It is

said that it takes 21 days to form a new habit, so you should expect that applying the new ideas, and the basic principles of addressing your endometriosis naturally, will take time. It may take some weeks to form a routine that works for you, depending on your level of commitment and economic resources. Remember that a natural approach to endometriosis is not a 'quick fix', but a permanent lifestyle change. It may have taken you years, if not decades, of being around toxins to get into this state so it will not be a quick route out either. Be realistic, be kind to yourself and above all, start to believe in yourself.

It took me about three to four months to really see and feel a recognisable difference. It then took my body a few years to be fully energised to where I am now. Still to this day, I am continuously making adjustments where and when I need to. For some women, the healing process may be faster than mine – after all, I did have other conditions on top of endometriosis. I had also experienced those other conditions for a very long time, and I was the guinea pig for myself. I had to try everything out on myself firsthand and learn and research. You are lucky as you get to walk in my footsteps and only have to follow the guidelines in this book and implement the suggestions. Although some people achieve relief quickly, for others it takes a bit longer. The key is never to give up.

The principles of reconnecting to your body and learning to listen to it take time to implement. Sometimes, it can help to focus on what mental adjustments we need to make to increase our awareness of belief systems, as we are reluctant to 'give up' food or a product that is making us ill. There may be some questioning of beliefs about who is responsible for your body.

Ultimately, we are responsible for our bodies. No one else is. We have to change our attitude towards our bodies as we are the ones who have to live in them after doctors or surgeons have finished 'tinkering' with them. You may want to stop and ask yourself this: if the body is always wanting to regenerate and repair itself, then what is stopping it? Put on your detective hat. Remember – anything worth having does not come easily and this goes for your health too.

It is time to let go of what is holding you back, reclaim your power and follow your instincts to get out of pain.

Get on the right natural path – the EndoBoss® path.

If you do, you will see a reduction in, then elimination of, pain. You will regain energy and vitality. You will be able to live your best life!

These new habits will be the difference between you remaining in pain, with a hot water bottle attached to your abdomen for the rest of your life, or breaking free and moving forward.

I aim to get you living the life you deserve to live; pain-free, and fulfilling the destiny you were sent here for. Endometriosis sufferers deserve to be able to enjoy their lives before their time here passes. So many women with endometriosis have spent their whole lives just surviving; now it is time to live and thrive. All you have to do is just take the first small step, then the next. Before you know it, your body will thank you.

The level of pain and symptoms in your body will determine the level of changes that you need to make in your life. For results to be seen, changes will need to be made. Do not expect health to magically 'rain down' upon you.

To see results, you need to take ACTION.

When you commit to these routines, you will reap the benefits. These new routines changed my life. And yes, annoyingly at times I had to make changes I was reluctant to make. Yes, it was hard at times. But I am loving being where I am now. I am still pain-free and have no pelvic pain or endometriosis and adenomyosis symptoms. I am also now free of mitochondria dysfunction, CFS and thyroid issues.

The changes I made and the bumps in the road that I had to go over were worth it – they were necessary to get to where I am now. It took me 14 years of extensive research and experimentation to learn the principles in this book. Now you have all that I learned in your hands, and this will allow you to take control of your body and your life.

Expect that you may get a little frustrated or despondent, and you may even 'fall off the wagon' at times. If you do fall off, just like falling off a horse or a bike, get back on (without beating yourself up) and keep on going.

I encourage you to set yourself realistic goals and also to have the odd 'treat'. When you have your 'treat', allow yourself one of your favourite foods – it can be anything from a chocolate bar to a packet of crisps (make sure they have NO wheat in them though). Try to get the healthiest version of your treat too as then it will minimise any ill effects (like a bar of dark chocolate made with lots of cocoa and very little sugar).

Assuming you have achieved your intermediate goals, for example something like replacing your toxic washing powder with non-toxic organic coconut-based washing powder, then have a 'treat' to reward yourself without guilt. Never deny yourself any type of food as you may find you crave it more. Just negotiate with yourself, set a goal, achieve it, and then treat yourself. This philosophy has worked wonders for my children and me. Then, after you have had the treat, notice how your body feels after eating it and then get back on the wagon. Remember, you want to leave the pain behind, so recommit to yourself, and keep recommitting to yourself, to getting back on the path to healing and a pain-free body.

Like going through the layers of an onion, the principles of this *Endometriosis Naturally* book is about helping you to identify which of the many potential sources are increasing your inflammation and pain. Expect to become quite adept at establishing, discovering, and unfolding which sources are causing you pain.

It is time to take back control and responsibility of your body and your life.

Here are the 12 basic principles:

1) Test for Nutritional and Digestive Imbalances

If you have the financial resources to do so, get a blood, hair, and saliva analysis test for nutritional deficiencies. Ask your doctor to test for B12 and ferritin iron blood levels. Consider doing the home test for stomach acid using the bicarbonate of soda test.

2) Natural Progesterone and Estradiol (Estrogen) Levels

Consider getting a saliva test done for estradiol, progesterone, and cortisol. Supplement with natural bioidentical progesterone cream to correct progesterone deficiencies and hormonal imbalances. Check over ingredients as you are looking for a bioidentical progesterone cream and ensure it contains no fragrances, perfumes, phytoestrogens, or chemicals like parabens and SLS.

3) Avoid All Wheat Products

If you only try one thing from this book, make sure you try cutting out wheat flour from your diet for a minimum period of three months. Look for items containing possible hidden wheat on the label – for example dextrin (e.g. maltodextrin), modified starch, monosodium glutamate, malt, wheat germ flour, spelt flour, wheat germ oil, wheat pectin, wheat glucose syrup, thickening, couscous, semolina, cereal filler, rusk, bran, soy sauce, lagers, and beers.

4) You Are What You Eat

Eating healthy, fresh, organic fruit and vegetables plus grass-fed, hormone-free, free-range meat, poultry, and fish is essential and more details about diet will follow. Try goat's milk or coconut milk as an alternative to cow's milk. Fresh line caught fish (but not from a fish farm) – frozen fish from the supermarket is inexpensive, easy to store in bulk and super easy to cook. My favourite meal is cooking fresh fish in coconut oil with some garlic and herbs. Although, be mindful that some herbs may be inflammatory to some women, contrary to what some claims made about them online.

Nuts and seeds are excellent sources of protein, as are beans and pulses. Some women do well to exclude dairy from their diet, whilst others are ok consuming it. Take your time to establish if your body is reacting to any foods by keeping a food diary. I advise keeping a record of what you eat and how you feel, along with any physical reactions after you have eaten it.

5) Stomach Acid Test

Remember to test if you have enough hydrochloric acid in your stomach by doing the simple home bicarbonate of soda test. Take good quality digestive enzymes with every meal. You can eat all the good food in the world, but if you are unable to breakdown and digest the food, it will all be in vain. Fully absorbing your food, and the elimination of waste regularly will be covered in later chapters too. To replenish your 'good' bacteria in your bowel, you may also want to consider taking an acidophilus supplement.

Nutrients from your food are absorbed from your small bowel, through the lining and into your bloodstream. However, if the body is in a constant state of stress (in 'flight or fight' mode), the digestive tract stops functioning. Food consumed may not be broken down properly as digestive juices produced in the stomach (hydrochloric acid) may not be present. This means that undigested, unbroken down pieces of food may enter the intestinal tract, causing irritation and inflammation like irritable bowel syndrome (IBS).

6) Increase Protein Intake (Protein shake)

If pain has dampened your appetite and you are struggling to eat solid foods, it is essential that you 'drink' your daily nutrients and calories. If you are not consuming at least 1,500-2,000 calories a day, you will feel weak and struggle to do even the most basic of tasks. Your organs require nutrition and fuel to carry out even the most essential bodily functions. Remember that it is best to avoid synthetic products like Quorn (as it is an edible fungus) and tofu (which is made from soybeans).

Increase your protein consumption to around 1.5g of protein per kilogram of body weight (about 90g grams a day) and aim to have a protein shake every morning. Within one hour of waking, make your protein shake consisting of a pint of water/plant milk (e.g. coconut milk), two tablespoons of rice or pea organic protein powder (make sure it is good quality and not full of fillers and sugar/sweeteners), crush two good quality multivitamin and mineral tablets (like Solgar) or use rice-based multivitamin and mineral powder, and some 'Macro Greens'. One teaspoon of Macro Greens is the equivalent of five portions of fruit and vegetables. You may also want to invest in a juicer to start juicing your organic vegetables and fruits.

7) Correct Your Nutritional Deficiencies
Take a good quality multivitamin and mineral supplement every day. Try to get even more vitamins from eating plenty of nutrient-dense foods like vegetables and nuts. Heavy, prolonged bleeding and blood clots can make a lot of endometriosis woman deficient in iron. Ask your doctor to check your ferritin iron levels and correct any nutritional imbalances.

8) Remove Toxins and Estrogen Mimickers
Swap all plastics for ceramic and glassware. Stop cooking food in plastic and stop using the microwave. Instead, get cooking in the oven using ceramic. Swap out hair, make-up, personal and household products that contain chemicals, parabens or SLSs. Swap chemical-laden washing powders for coconut-based products instead, but again check the labels for any unwanted chemicals. Be aware that nail varnish

and hair dyes are particularly toxic. Peel all non-organic fruit and vegetables. Cease the use of all synthetic and chemical drugs, including painkillers if possible.

9) Natural Aromatase Inhibitors

Support your body's natural healing mechanisms that metabolise excess estrogens by using supplements like natural aromatase inhibitors such as DIM, myomin, pycnogenol or I3C.

10) Systemic Enzyme Therapy

Use natural enzyme supplements such as the well-studied serrapeptase or nattokinase that have anti-inflammatory effects and can help dissolve, reduce, and prevent blood clots, adhesions, and cysts. Use digestive enzymes with every meal to ensure you get the maximum nutritional benefit from your food.

11) Befriend Your Body

You are beginning a journey to learn about yourself and befriend your body. You will learn how to listen to your body and how to interpret the signs and messages it is giving you. Up until now, your body may have just been this 'vessel' to carry your head around. You may have even hated your body for causing you so much pain and distress.

Start by just noticing the people in your life who are energy-draining, energy-neutral or energy-giving. You might be surprised at what you notice – but do not feel guilty, whatever the discovery is, even if it is a family member or close friend, make a point of noticing it. Listen to your 'gut' instincts as your body is always trying to communicate with you. Listening to your body will become very empowering for you as you progress through the principles. The strengthening of this relationship with your body will be a focus during these next few months.

12) Journalling

As you are recovering from endometriosis, you may start to re-examine some areas of your life. An excellent way to increase your awareness of what works (and what does not work) for you is to write a journal or diary entry every day. In Julia Cameron's book, *The Artist Way*, she refers to this journalling process as 'The Morning Pages'. It is a way to record your thoughts, feelings, self-pity, anxieties, fears, and hopes – really whatever comes to mind. There is no wrong way to write your journal, but I would recommend you do it for at least 12 weeks. Every morning upon awakening, take 20-30 minutes to write down the first things that come to mind on three sides of an A5 page; do not worry if all you write is, "I don't know what to write!"

Some mornings even though I had not even slept, I wrote anyway. I wrote when I was sad, depressed, anxious, or just plain puffed out with it all. I wrote even when all I felt was just plain negative, or if I was ecstatically positive. I wrote every single day, no matter what, and you need to as well. However, you might be surprised how you feel AFTER you have written out all that is going on in your head. A word of caution, though: keep these words private to you for now. This is about you and only you. You are writing a diary to record your progress, hear your inner voice, and monitor reductions in pain and symptoms.

If writing on paper does not feel safe or private enough, then there are some great mobile apps for journalling online, or you can use platforms like notes or Evernote. Journalling was, and still is, an excellent way for me to see and mark my progress. I understand that you may think you will never forget this period in your life, with all the pain and suffering you are enduring, but you will – because I did!

Only when I went back and reread my old diaries did I realise the progress I had made and just how much pain I was in – but also just how wonderful it is to be out of pain now. I tell everyone I meet to journal – even those without endometriosis – as it is just so powerful. Both my son and my daughter have benefitted and gained so much from journalling as well.

Journalling is a great way to hear your dreams for the future, and to listen to what is within your heart and soul. That little voice has been drowned out by pain, perpetual worry, busyness, thinking about others, and background anxiety. Now is the time to think about yourself and your future. So let me explain a little more the background and benefits to journalling in the next chapter.

Chapter 22 -

The Joy of Journalling

* * *

Journalling is like whispering to one's self and listening at the same time

— *Mina Murray*

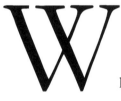hen it was first suggested to me to put pen on paper

and write across the page in a journal, I was very resistant.

You see, when I was in my early teenage years, I had kept a small journal and made some loose notes about my dreams. However, I came back from school one day, and my mother had it in her hand. She scowled as she waved it in front of my face with judgement and scorn pouring from her tongue.

To this day, it is a little unclear what was so terrible about what I had written, but I do know that I never wrote privately like that again.

That is until I read the wonderful book called *The Artist's Way* by Julia Cameron.

I have read many books throughout the years of this journey, and each one holds a special place in my heart and provided me with healing in different ways. With Julia's book, her encouragement to write in the morning, upon awakening, was life-changing and I shall always feel grateful for her writing that book.

So I encourage you to journal every morning as you wake up. It is natural to feel some resistance to journalling and pouring out one's own private thoughts and feelings on paper.

There may be this thought of, "What if someone reads it?" or "What if they think me crazy or mad?"

Keep It Private
Well, I do suggest that you keep what you write down private. Do not be tempted to share with a partner, husband, friends, or family. What you write down is personal to you and is not to be disclosed. If you find a partner or family member is becoming more interested or curious about your new writing habit, then instead of sharing that you are writing about thoughts and feelings, say that you are only writing about your physical symptoms.

I find that people are not so interested in people writing about physical ailments, yet may become quite nosey about emotions, thoughts and feelings. So be careful to keep your journal private, under lock and key if necessary.

Embrace Your Emotions

What you are looking to do every morning is to write all your thoughts and feelings and emotions onto paper. Let the ink pour out and stain the paper with any fear, worry, anxiety, dread, depression, anger, sadness, negativity, or apprehension.

You will notice resistance to doing so – perhaps because societies around the globe promote only positivity of thought all the time.

Of course, we all seek to be that glass half-filled type of person.

Yet, the reality is that the pressure to be super-positive all the time can make you feel like a failure, especially if you dare to have one negative or sad thought or feeling.

Remember that it is natural to have sad days, bad days, down days, and flare days.

Days that you feel like giving up and throwing in the towel.

Days that you feel like the world is against you.

Days of despair when you feel like your body is a wreck and you doubt if it will ever get better.

However, an interesting shift occurs when you write down thoughts and unpleasant feelings on to paper. Believe it or not they actually lessen, dissolve, and disappear, allowing for the pleasant thoughts, feelings and aspirations and your own internal guidance to appear.

The enormous amount of energy that is required to try and suppress negative or unpleasant feelings is underestimated.

As a woman with endometriosis, you have already endured much pain and suffering and now is the time to allow some gentle processing of the past and the present to begin.

Flow of Consciousness

The real purpose of putting pen to paper is to learn the art of letting go of what and who is not important to you (or indeed be toxic and harmful to you).

By encouraging the writing of your flow of consciousness, you get everything that is stuck in your mind onto paper and develop a habit of 'just noticing'.

You will learn to 'just notice' your natural fluctuation in feelings and emotions.

You will learn to 'just notice' who upsets you, who makes you cry or who makes you angry. Please do not feel ashamed of feeling the emotion of anger. Anger is an amazing emotion that tells you somebody has tried to disrespect you or your boundaries. Learn to listen to the feeling and put your thoughts on paper.

It is critical to allow your most genuine thoughts, beliefs, and feelings to be dispersed onto the page. Over time your resistance to writing will disappear and your writing will become a joyful and truly authentic experience. Journalling will help you to deeply connect to the beautiful and more vulnerable parts that lie hidden within you.

This is why it is imperative that no one is permitted to read your journal.

Untapping Your Inner Genius

Sometimes secrets, events, or experiences in the past, that I have tried to stop thinking about, are poured onto paper with a huge wave of relief. Writing has allowed me to gently grieve certain stages of my life. The years of isolation, disability, mistreatment, and lost dreams have been given the time and respect to pass.

Try to focus on keeping your hand moving across the page and remind yourself that all you need to do is keep moving forward and write down the thoughts and chatter in your head.

Some mornings my mind is like a chirpy chatty monkey or like a blue-bottle fly bouncing off the walls of a room.

When my mind is whirling around, I just write as fast as I can. This allows the transfer of my thoughts on to paper so that I can have greater clarity for the day ahead.

This process is helping you to retrain your brain to manage your mind.

Over time you will recognise the joy of journalling and welcome the pages like a safe and kind friend with whom you can share your innermost thoughts, feelings, and emotions.

There is research to back up the claims of how writing on paper every day helps reduce anxiety, stress, and even trauma.[37]

Writing Your Way Back To You

I do morning pages every single day, no matter what. It does not matter how I feel, where I am or what is happening in my life. I recognise the deep value in journalling and how it positively helps me emotionally and even physically disperse the tension in my muscles.

I know when I am about to grow personally or spiritually as that is when I may feel resistance to journalling.

However, I pick up my pen and journal, notice resistance and write anyway.

As Julia Cameron, the author of *The Artist Way* states lovingly, "make the morning pages non-negotiable".

Just write your way back to you.

Chapter 23 -

Relaxation, Mindfulness & Meditation

* * *

Quiet The Mind & The Soul Will Speak

— Budha

As part of my research, I remember reading that deep

relaxation, mindfulness, and meditation may help with a vast range of illnesses, along with psychological and emotional issues such as depression. If I am honest, I remember being somewhat cynical.

Firstly, I was not even sure what relaxation meant. Relaxation was what other people did. I was always filled with too much guilt, stress, and anxiety to sit still and relax. The idea of mindfulness and meditation all seemed a little too 'different', 'out there' and 'new age' to me at the start.

The dictionary definition of mindfulness, for example, is "*the quality or state of being conscious or aware of something*" and "*a mental state achieved by focusing one's awareness on the present moment, while calmly acknowledging and accepting one's feelings, thoughts, and bodily sensations, used as a therapeutic technique".*

However, I continued to read and had my mind and brain blown away by the countless studies and experiments that validated this simple process. The positive effects of mindfulness are profound for people who practice it. The practice is still relatively new in the Western world, but studies share the impact it has had in the relatively short period it has been around. Mindfulness and meditation are scientifically proven to be a viable alternative to current treatments like antidepressants.[38]

Mindfulness meditation therapy may also help to manage pain and reduce stress, and the great thing about it is that anyone can do it. Mindfulness meditation therapy is a very natural and safe way to treat and recover yourself naturally.

When mindfulness meditation was first suggested to me, I thought I might have to sit cross-legged on top of a hill, making a humming sound. It felt like a slightly preposterous practice. I have to share that this type of meditation has been hugely beneficial to me, and when I have had a session, I equate it to feeling like I have been recharged after being plugged into an electrical socket.

In mindfulness meditation, the first thing it does is change the brainwave into a relaxing and restful state; referred to as theta. Once this practice is underway, you may notice how it slows down your brain rhythm, your heart rate, metabolism, breathing rate, and even has been shown to lower blood pressure too. This theta state can be achieved quite easily by simply focusing all of your attention on your breath, i.e. breathing in for seven seconds, holding for four, and then gently pushing out your breath slowly for eleven seconds.

Natural painkillers in your body called endorphins are released into your system, leaving you in a peaceful state of mind, observing your surroundings without forming judgments or thinking about anything else. Like with anything new, it takes time to develop the techniques and skill. But it is worth persevering.

Mindfulness meditating may need some practice, especially if you are not used to doing it. You may find that thoughts are rushing in like a jumpy, chirpy monkey! However, after some time and practice, you should find that you can clear your mind of thoughts and induce a comfortable, deeper relaxed state.

Mindfulness meditation therapy is widely practised nowadays, even in seemingly unlikely places like the offices of Wall Street. It has been shown to relieve nervous system problems such as headaches, anxiety, stroke, depression, epilepsy, and multiple sclerosis. For women who suffer from excruciating endometriosis pain, mindfulness meditation therapy has been proven to help improve the immune system. It can also help you to 'just notice' your thoughts like clouds in the sky passing you by during periods of stress or anxiety.

Another great thing about mindfulness meditation therapy is that it has no adverse side effects, only good ones. You do not need to spend any money because it is free. As a beginner, all you need is intent, a lot of determination and a little place of peace and quiet to start to practise calming down your active conscious mind. Try the many different mobile applications for guided meditations available, as well as tracks on music streaming platforms like Spotify or iTunes (many of which are free), which encourage you to lie back, enjoy, and relax.

Do not worry about 'doing it right'; there is no right or wrong way. If you sit up or lie down or even fall asleep, do not worry, as it is better for you and your body because you fall into a deeper relaxed state of sleep. Little by little, you will allow your mind and your body as a whole to get into that slow, gentle rhythm and reach a relaxing state of calm. There is no better feeling in this world than the meditative level of calm and peace. When you attain that, you will ultimately learn to hear that little quiet voice within yourself. That voice, along with this book, can guide you towards being finally, victoriously free from endometriosis.

Chapter 24 -

Toxic People & Naysayers

* * *

"Just as there is Nothing Wrong in Avoiding a Flame that Burns You, There is Nothing Wrong in Avoiding People Who Hurt You"

– Wendy K Laidlaw

I am hoping by this point in the book that you are starting to

feel that small ember of hope get a bit bigger and brighter.

I am praying that a small part of you is saying softly in your ear, *"What if?"*

"What if, because this approach worked for Wendy, and all these other women around the globe, then maybe, just maybe, it might work for me too?"

If you are having that faint thought, I am delighted – because that is the essence of my book and my intention.

I intend to ignite that hope and faith. Those two crucial elements you need as a woman with endometriosis:

- Hope in your body's ability to heal.

- Faith in your ability to be determined enough to make it happen.

I regularly remind to my EndoBoss® students that this is not an easy journey. Nor is it a quick one either.

But it is a worthy one.

It takes time for the cells in your body to repair and regenerate, and I think this is the point where again I remind you that it is a journey.

A journey to get to understand your body (what it likes and does not like) as well as your mind, soul, and spirit. The journey may be challenging at times, but I promise it is so worth it to get to the other side.

I would love to share with you the story about 'The Beggar & The Box'.

Back in Roman times, there was a bedraggled old beggar who sat in his tattered clothes on a dilapidated box by the side of the road. He had sat there for many, many years.

Day in and day out, swarms of strangers would pass him on their way into the nearby town, and the beggar did what all beggars do, which was to ask for money.

The strangers would look at him with disdain and take a wide berth to avoid him.

One day a traveller with a kind face was passing on his way towards town, and the beggar shouted over to him, "Kind sir, please would you give me some money?"

Approaching him cautiously, the traveller said, "I'm so sorry, I don't have any money to spare."

The two men then started to have a conversation, and the traveller asked what misfortune had befallen the beggar to have him begging by the roadside.

The beggar explained how he had lost his family due to disease, and how he had lost his land to neighbouring bullies a few years ago.

Then the traveller inquired, "So, I am curious about your box that you are sitting on – tell me more about the story behind that."

"What about my box?" the beggar replied.

"Well, what's in it?" questioned the traveller.

The beggar responded, "I don't know – it's just an old box I found here many years ago, and I've been sitting on it ever since."

Persistent in his inquiry, the traveller once again questioned about what was in the box.

The beggar replied, "I've never looked."

The traveller said, "Why not?"

"Because there is nothing there!" the beggar howled back impatiently.

The traveller said, "Well, let's take a look, shall we?"

Finally, to appease the traveller's insistence, the beggar stood up, shakily and stiffly, and turned around to observe the box.

The beggar bent down and as he began to lift up the lid of the old wooden box, he let out a gasp.

"What on earth do I see? Do my eyes deceive me?"

Amazingly, within the box, there was a treasure trove of gold coins filled to the brim.

The beggar had been sitting on his box of 'treasure' for years and never even knew what lay within.

And, with his inquisition satisfied, off the traveller went.

The moral of the story is: 'What treasure are you sitting on?' and 'What is it going to take for you to open it?'

I invite you to look inside of yourself and see the untold treasure that lies within; and that you did not know you possessed.

When we start this new journey, I may be that stranger who is asking you to 'look inside' of yourself and trust your inner wisdom and gut instincts.

Once you decide to embark on this journey, you may encounter some people who are unhappy with you starting on your new pathway.

I call these disgruntled people 'the naysayers'. People who are energy vampires – constantly negative and complaining yet doing nothing themselves about their misery.

You, however, *are* doing something about yours, and this may threaten them in some peculiar way.

You may expect your friends and family to be happy for you, and to support you for trying to take back control and power on a new pathway. You then might feel confused when they criticise and chastise you for what you are doing.

My grandfather used to say, "The birds always pick at the ripest cherries." So be wary of those who are not supportive of your new endeavour.

One of the most confusing stages was when I approached my local GP and specialist surgeon with great glee and excitement about my improvements within a few months. I eagerly explained what I was doing and how it was working.

Naively, I had expected them to be supportive and happy for me – I even thought they might be encouraging cheerleaders, wishing me well.

That did not happen.

Instead, the opposite happened, and it shocked me.

I made a conscious decision early on to only to engage with people who supported me, and there were few.

I wrote down a list of the toxic people – family, friends, and colleagues – and made sure that I limited my engagement with them, and told them little or nothing about what I was doing.

Some part of me recognised that I had to protect my soul and my spirit from people who were not supportive or encouraging of my intentions to do it naturally.

Start to notice who are your supporters – who are rooting for you and cheering you on – and make sure to spend extra quality time around them, or engaging with them.

It could make all the difference to your health as you discover the wealth that lies within yourself!

Chapter 25 -

Begin Your Natural Journey

* * *

Don't be afraid to take a big step if one is indicated; you can't cross a chasm in two small jumps
— David Lloyd George

From all of this flood of information, I can safely say that

all who suffer from endometriosis should treat it like a fire. The fire stays alive for as long as there is heat, fuel to burn, and oxygen to breathe. Take away any one of those three elements, and the fire will go out. In the same fashion, we should also take away the various elements that endometriosis feeds on. By doing so, we are depriving it of its source of life, and eventually it will simply die out, just like fire.

Now, we know that endometriosis is caused by the growth of endometrial-like tissue outside of the uterus, when it should be lining the inside. Medical experts have not entirely determined why this happens and what causes the tissue to grow outside of its natural environment.

The principles behind how I ended my endometriosis naturally involve addressing endometriosis at a cellular, deep root level. Conventional medicine misses several stages of endometriosis and tries to manage the symptoms rather than identify and eliminate the underlying causes. Medical treatment does not address endometriosis naturally. Painkillers, drugs, and surgery merely keep you in an endless, deteriorating cycle of chronic debilitating pain, hormonal imbalances, enzyme disruption, organ malfunctions, and other awful side effects. The Heal Endometriosis Naturally process stops infertility, eliminates pain, restores energy, and mends the damage that has been caused to your body by the medical process.

We know that endometriosis is an estrogen-dominant condition and that a woman's body must maintain higher levels of progesterone to balance this out. Therefore, how do we avoid this hormone imbalance? We need to prevent estrogen levels from going up. The very first step to do this is to be very mindful of our environment.

As we have discussed in earlier chapters, estrogen can be found in just about anything, from plastics to cosmetics, to food, and much more. Check all of the things that you have around the house. Take a close look at the ingredients in your cosmetics, toilet-cleaning agents, dairy and food products.

If there are ingredients that are alien to you or if you cannot pronounce their names, chances are these can be harmful to you – and worse, may contain estrogen mimickers. Discard these things right away, if finances allow, to avoid further contamination. Package up all of the offending items in a box and donate them to a charity or a friend. If you cannot afford to replace them immediately, then do your best to reduce your usage and research the alternatives in advance.

I have mentioned that estrogen is also present in the food that we eat. This hormone is mostly found in processed food, from vegetable and grain farms heavily sprayed with pesticides, and from livestock heavily induced with growth hormones. Therefore, when you go out to shop for food, be sure to buy only the freshest fruits, vegetables, fish, and meat. For the meat, try to investigate if the source is wild, free-range, hormone-free, and grass-fed.

In the UK, many online companies provide fantastic unprocessed, organic, hormone and pesticide-free food, and will deliver it directly to your door – many at surprisingly low prices too, so please take advantage of them.

If you decide enough is enough, and you are going to commit to getting yourself out of pain, then from this point on you need to discipline yourself to have the patience to prepare your food. If you are a busy person and your work demands a lot of your time during the day, then you need to devise a time management plan to include food preparation in your daily schedule. Make time to think ahead. This is where I fell initially and made it harder on myself – by not planning ahead. Because you are buying nothing but fresh food, this needs to be prepared and cooked as soon as possible to avoid spoilage.

Indulge yourself with protein-rich diets. Remember if you are in so much pain and you are struggling to eat solid food, make your protein shake every morning and pour in all of that goodness to assist your body in its healing. Ample concentrations of protein in our body keep all of our vital internal organs healthy. Once we attain that proper and healthy balance of food intake, we make our liver happy. Moreover, if our liver is working correctly, we will no longer worry about our estrogen levels going up.

We need to keep our bodies active, but only if we are able. We should try and find time to engage in some small amount of physical activity, even if it is only a short walk or sitting outside for 20 minutes per day. When you are out of pain, yoga, Pilates, or swimming are gentle and supportive ways to strengthen your body.

For some of us, the idea of making a change may seem like a daunting and arduous task. When we are in constant, chronic, and persistent low-level pain, it can be hard to function on a daily basis, let alone think about what to eat, then have to go out, purchase it and finally cook it. If you are in a lot of pain with no appetite, I encourage you, at the very least, have one protein shake every day, as previously mentioned. You will be amazed at how even that one small change can make a big difference.

You will now have to commit to making a complete lifestyle change. Go out and shop around for everything that is 'green', paraben-free, SLS free, organic, or made from natural ingredients. There are natural alternatives for cosmetics too. As for cleaning products, many do-it-yourself alternatives use only natural ingredients. The internet is full of many wonderful suggestions.

Our body is not a separate entity from our minds, and we are surrounded in our lives with toxic environments and pollutants. Our body is a byproduct of our environment – it is affected by what comes in, on, and around it.

What we are looking to do here is to take small steps, and make one small change at a time.

Equally, it can be tempting to go rushing in with great enthusiasm and want to do everything and change it immediately. Please do not do that either. All that will happen is you may get overwhelmed, confused, and frustrated, then grind to an exhausted halt. If you make too many changes too quickly, you will find it harder to adapt, and then the changes are likely to be unsustainable. You are looking to make lifestyle changes that last forever. This is not a quick, temporary program that will end and have you better within a few weeks.

My advice is to get comfortable and adapt to each change – after all, you will be living with these changes for many months, years and maybe even the rest of your life. As a minimum though, you are in this for the next five to six months or so and hopefully beyond, so pace yourself for the long haul and give yourself realistic goals.

Many times, I zoomed down a path of treatment at 100 miles per hour like I was the old cartoon character Road Runner on speed, bursting with enthusiasm, prepared to fully embrace my new find. Then after a short time, I got stuck, hit a wall, burnt myself out and lost direction.

This is where my motto 'Slow is Fast' came in. I learned to integrate the new principles and ideas slowly but – most importantly – to bring back into BALANCE all areas of my body and my life. Before, when I was in chronic pain, my life was forever out of balance, as were my estrogen and progesterone levels. Balance is a very delicate thing and is different for everyone. But nevertheless, balance is key.

I was in a very distressed and painful state five years ago and naturally I, like most women, wished for a magic wand to come along and give me a 'quick fix' instantly. However, life does not work like that. I learnt that it had taken me a long time to get into the condition I was in, and it was going to take quite some time to get the balance back into my body. I also learned that when I tried to rush the change, it ended up taking me longer. Consistency and persistence are the keys!

Every woman is unique and different – therefore, each recovery journey will be personal to the individual woman. However, there are some commonalities and areas that we can assess to help us get started, on track and ultimately to get you out of pain, naturally.

It takes time to see the results. When I get asked, "Wendy, how long before I can start to see results?" my answer is always the same. I saw a 50% reduction in pain within eight weeks. Thus, continuing to follow the principles resulted in the total elimination of pain within five to six months. But everyone is different, so what works for one woman may not work for another.

You may take more or less time to heal, depending on your medical history. You have the basic principles and roadmap now. Just keep on the road, apply the basic principles and never, ever, give up.

Later in this book, I will also give you a link to further resources especially for EndoBoss® Beginners (like you), to help you begin on your healing journey, as well as detail the additional support options that are available to you.

You will be becoming your own detective about your body, learning to listen and notice how your body is responding to the principles. You will learn to make adjustments, or move to the next step when your body is ready.

But most importantly, be kind, compassionate, and gentle on yourself. The pain of endometriosis has beaten you up enough.

And as Winston Churchill so eloquently said -

"Never give in. Never give in. Never, never, never, never — in nothing, great or small, large or petty — never give in, except to convictions of honour and good sense."

Chapter 26

Support

* * *

Destiny is not a matter of chance; it is a matter of choice. It is not something to be waited for but rather something to be achieved.

– William Jennings Bryan

S upport is available in many forms if you get stuck or feel like

you need a morale boost; but please, no matter what, do NOT ever give up hope. Join a positive and supportive online group or forum to reassure yourself you are not alone, ideally one that supports a natural approach to full health. On our Resources page, you can find a link to join our HealEndometriosisNaturallyBook Group on Facebook.

Expect to be frustrated, impatient, and have the odd set back at times. That is entirely normal. But do not lose hope. Have abject faith in you and your body. If you have a flare day, bad day, sad day, or down day, acknowledge that it will pass and get back on the path again, recommit to yourself and keep moving forward. Have faith that your body wants to repair and regenerate itself and you have the power to do that. I believe in your body's ability to heal if you give it the right environment and ingredients – and of course, remove the poisons that are preventing it from healing.

If you hit a period of non-progression, then go back to step one and reread the information in this book. Ask yourself what you might have missed or are missing? What has 'sneaked' back into your diet? What is new in your household products, or personal products, or stress that you had not noticed? Are you taking adequate supplements, eating enough protein or have you had a hormone test done? Have you tried natural progesterone cream (or 'balancing cream' some manufacturers call it now)? Or have you tried the systemic enzyme therapy or natural aromatase inhibitors? Are you getting enough sleep and drinking enough fluids? Check what works for you, keep listening to your body and keep a record of your progress in your journal.

One day I would love to hear and read about your journey to a pain-free body and putting your endometriosis naturally into remission – your journey from surviving and struggling in pain, to thriving and talking about your success. Then maybe apply to train as an EndoBoss® Coach or Endometriosis Health Coach with me to help spread this message of hope and healing. We all have a responsibility to share the positive pathway and it is my mission to share to millions of women, so we can educate, empower, and inspire them to end their endometriosis naturally.

If you feel you need more one-on-one support, then consider applying for a place on our EndoBoss® Academy online program. Please contact the EndoBoss® team at:
Support@HealEndometriosisNaturally.ZohoDesk.com

You are not alone and resources, webinars, programs, and training is available online at:
https://www.healendometriosisnaturally.com

Sending you all of my healing love and hugs,

To your health!

Wendy xx

Chapter 27

Meal Options

* * *

We are what we repeatedly do. Excellence then is not an act,
but a habit

— Aristotle.

T here is so much confusion out on the internet about what

to eat if you have endometriosis. As I mentioned earlier, the 'Endometriosis Diet' has many variations and suggestions.

The only real way to know what works for your body is to pay attention to how your body feels when you eat a specific food. You know your body better than anyone. I followed the recommendations of the 'Stone Age Eating Habits' suggested by Dr Sarah Myhill, who helped me combat my CFS. It is super simple. It goes on the premise and ideology of following what our great, great ancestors predominately ate – i.e. plants, vegetables, fruits, nuts, and seeds and also occasionally meat (predominately chicken and fish).

This is what worked for me. If you are vegetarian or vegan, then remove any meats or animal products but do know that you will need to supplement your body with more protein shakes and amino acid supplements. Meat and eggs cause some confusion for women with endometriosis. I did not find chicken or fish or eggs (all of which were as fresh as possible, free-range, hormone-free, grass-fed) to be an inflammatory issue for me. Red meat, however, did not always agree with me, so I tend to avoid it unless is it hormone-free, antibiotic-free and grass fed. Equally, the only way to know if these foods are inflammatory to you is to keep a regular food journal. Your body will tell you within 20 minutes to an hour if it has an issue with these foods. The secret is to learn to pay attention to how your body feels, reacts and responds.

What helped me on my journey with diet and creating healthy eating habits was to ask myself; "*Would my great great great grandmother have eaten this?*" – i.e. checking if it was highly processed, artificial or 'fake', or was it filled with additives, preservatives, antibiotics, hormones and pesticides?

I had been unaware of the impact of food on my endometriosis in the past and did not give a thought to what I ate and how it affected my body. But now I do. Being mindful of what I eat and how it affects me means the difference between being in pain or not, and keeping endometriosis and adenomyosis and cysts and adhesions in remission. This new relationship with my body is why I have been entirely pain-free in my pelvis for years now.

There are many wonderful wheat-free and gluten-free cookbooks out now, (and I have my own called *Heal Endometriosis Naturally Cookbook with 101 Recipes* available on Amazon) but the central theme you are looking to follow is 'fresh is best' and go 'Stone Age'.

At the start, keep your eating super, super simple. Then, later on, experiment further with simple and basic ingredients like free-range organic eggs, to begin with – become creative, making omelettes or pancakes or even have a super simple boiled egg.

There was an advertising slogan used during the 1950s and 1960s by the United Kingdom's Egg Marketing Board which said: *"Go to work on an egg!"*

Eggs are very cost-effective and in addition to being packed full of nutrition, eggs are usually easy to digest compared to some other high-protein foods– that is, as long as they are from free-range, outdoor reared, happy chickens!

Clearly if you have an allergy to eggs then avoid them completely or if you have an intolerance then leave eating them for at least 12 weeks and introduce slowly and check in with your body's responses to it.

Below are some other ideas to help get you started and you will find more in my *Heal Endometriosis Naturally Cookbook with 101 Recipes* available on Amazon.

Breakfast Choices

- Rice or gluten-free oats low sugar cereal, with coconut or plant milk and berries (strawberries, raspberries, or blueberries).

- Rice flour tortillas, warmed, with scrambled eggs, chopped tomato, and melted goats cheese.

- Cream of rice with chopped almonds and coconut/plant milk.

- Omelettes with vegetables (like onions, peppers, and tomatoes) and cold meats like ham or chicken.

- Gluten-free porridge oats or rice flakes with chopped fruit, cinnamon, or agar/rice syrup.

- Organic fresh fruit like apples or pears, chopped.

- Homemade gluten & wheat-free rice flour pancakes with agar or rice syrup.

- Dairy-free yoghurt (such as brands called Coyo or Nush) layered with crushed oatcakes and berries.

- Goats cheese mixed and layered with berries.

- Mashed avocado with tuna on gluten-free bread.

- Hard-boiled eggs mixed with humous, served on toasted gluten-free bread.

- Bacon (free-range, hormone-free, dry-cured).

- Frozen fruit smoothies mixed with juiced green vegetables.

Lunch Choices

- Sliced free-range turkey with lettuce, tomato, and humous on warmed rice flour tortillas with baby carrots.

- Grilled sliced free-range chicken over mixed greens with red peppers, sliced tomato, broccoli florets, and chickpeas, served with oil and vinegar or gluten-free salad dressing.

- Toasted gluten-free bread with tuna fish made with red pepper humous or smashed avocado, chopped onion, sliced tomato, shredded lettuce, and chopped cucumber.

- Smoked salmon or tuna served over mixed greens with shredded carrots, chopped tomatoes, and cucumbers. Served with oil and vinegar, or your favourite gluten-free salad dressing, rice crackers, and lemon wedges.

- Ham and goats cheese on gluten-free toast with mustard and coleslaw.

- Grilled free-range chicken cutlet marinated in garlic, oil, and lemon, served over chopped rocket, spinach red onion and lettuce, with wheat-free Caesar dressing, chopped nuts, grapes, and grated goats cheese.

- Grilled, 5% fat free-range, grass fed sirloin burger with lettuce, tomato, sautéed onion, a wheat-free roll and either reduced sugar ketchup or humous. If available serve over a mixed salad with olive oil and/or soy-free dressing and/or wheat-free vinegar. (If wheat protein is contained in vinegar, the label will say so).

- Grilled free-range chicken marinated in garlic, herbs, oil, salt, and pepper, with mashed sweet potato and mixed veggies.

Dinner Choices

- Salmon baked with lemon and dill, served with brown rice and steamed green beans.

- Hardboiled egg, sliced, with steamed green beans, baby spinach, sliced cucumber, sliced tomato, and chickpeas with oil and vinegar or gluten-free salad dressing.

- Grilled free-range chicken cutlet marinated in garlic, oil, and onion powder, served with cooked brown rice, steamed broccoli, and mixed greens served with oil and vinegar or gluten-free salad dressing.

- Cooked kidney beans and brown rice added to chopped onions sautéed in olive oil with garlic, with chopped tomato and chopped red pepper. Served with a green salad and wheat-free dressing.

- Free-range steak with garlic, herb and onion powder sauce, served with steamed cauliflower and a medium baked potato with butter.

- Baked flounder cooked with chopped onions, tomatoes, cilantro, garlic, and onion powder, served with steamed spinach, rice, and a mixed green salad with sliced tomato and cucumber and oil and vinegar or wheat-free salad dressing.

- Free-range pork loin cut into two-inch cubes and placed on a skewer with chunks of pineapple, cherry tomatoes marinated in wheat-free dressing, grilled, and served with steamed broccoli and corn with butter.

- Roasted free-range chicken with carrots, potatoes, and onions, seasoned with garlic, onion powder, salt, pepper, and herbs.

- Grilled or baked free-range chicken, shrimp, or veal, placed in a casserole dish and topped with tomato sauce, goats cheese, served with gluten-free pasta.

- Brown rice or vegetable pasta with tomato sauce and chicken and a mixed green salad with favourite gluten-free dressing.

- Grilled shrimp over a mixed salad with baby potatoes and wheat-free salad dressing.

- Hand-pressed grass-fed, hormone-free hamburger or turkey burger, with onion and sliced tomato, home-made baked sweet potato fries, and green beans.

Snack Choices

- Organic fresh fruit

- Dairy-free yoghurt (Coyo or Nush)

- Green & Blacks 80% dark chocolate (in moderation)

- Organic carrots/cucumber with humous

- Goats cheese with dried fruit

- Frozen plant milk with a lollipop handle

- Rice cakes

- Oatcakes (gluten-free)

- Nuts

Some Ingredients to Avoid (although not a definitive list)

Wheat, maltodextrin, Atta, kamut, bulgur, matzo meal, couscous, modified wheat starch, dinkel (also known as spelt), seitan, durum, semolina, einkorn, emmer, farro, heirloom, wheat bran, fu wheat flour, graham flour, wheat germ, hydrolysed wheat protein, wheat starch and buckwheat.

Chapter 28

Xenoestrogens

* * *

Do it now

— Napoleon Hill

Minimise Your Exposure to Xenoestrogens:

FOOD

- Avoid all pesticides, herbicides, and fungicides.

- Choose organic, locally-grown and in-season foods.

- Peel non-organic fruits and vegetables.

- Buy hormone-free, grass fed, free-range meats and food products.

PLASTICS

- Reduce the use of plastics.

- Do not microwave food in plastic containers but use glass instead.

- Do not use plastic wrap/cling film to cover food for storing or microwaving.

- Use glass or ceramic whenever possible to store or cook food.

- Do not leave plastic containers that contain food or drinking water in the sun.

- Throw away a plastic water container if it has been heated up.

HOUSEHOLD PRODUCTS

- Use chemical-free, coconut based, biodegradable laundry and household cleaning products.

- Choose chlorine-free products and unbleached paper products (tampons, menstrual pads, toilet paper, paper towels, coffee filters).

- Use a filter jug, chlorine filter on shower heads and filter drinking water. If possible install a household water filter that is able to filter all your water.

HEALTH AND BEAUTY PRODUCTS

- Avoid creams and cosmetics that have parabens, SLS and stearalkonium chloride.

- Reduce your exposure to nail polish and nail polish removers.

- Reduce the use of perfumes and use naturally based fragrances, such as essential oils.

- Use chemical-free, paraben-free, and SLS-free soaps.

- Use fluoride-free toothpaste.

- Read the labels on condoms and diaphragm gels.

POISONOUS NAMES TO LOOK OUT FOR:

CHEMICALS

- Skincare products – 4-Methyl benzylidene camphor (4-MBC).

- Sunscreen lotions – Benzophenone.

- All the parabens in body and face creams referred to as methylparaben, ethylparaben, propylparaben and butylparaben, which are commonly used as preservatives.

INDUSTRIAL PRODUCTS AND PLASTICS

- Bisphenol A (monomer for polycarbonate plastic and epoxy resin; antioxidant in plasticizers).

- Phthalates (plasticizers).

- DEHP (plasticizer for PVC).

- Polybrominated biphenyl ethers (PBDEs) (flame retardants used in plastics, foams, building materials, electronics, furnishings, motor vehicles).

- Polychlorinated biphenyls (PCBs).

FOOD

- Erythrosine/FD&C Red No. 3.

- Phenosulfothiazine (a red dye).

- Butylated hydroxyanisole/BHA (food preservative).

BUILDING SUPPLIES
- Pentachlorophenol (general biocide and wood preservative).

- Polychlorinated biphenyls/PCBs (in electrical oils, lubricants, adhesives, paints).

INSECTICIDES AND HERBICIDES
- Atrazine (weed killer).

- DDT (insecticide – banned in many countries nowadays).

- TCDD (2,3,7,8-Tetrachlorodibenzo-p-dioxin).

- Dieldrin (insecticide).

- Endosulfan (insecticide).

- Heptachlor (insecticide).

- Lindane/hexachlorocyclohexane (insecticide, used to treat lice and scabies).

- Methoxychlor (insecticide).

- Fenthion.

- Glyphosate-based herbicides like Roundup.

- Nonylphenol and derivatives (industrial surfactants; emulsifiers for emulsion polymerization; laboratory detergents; pesticides).

DRINKS

- Avoid carbonated or fizzy or sugary drinks.

- Sweeteners like fructose, sucralose and aspartame.

- Saccharin.

- Coffee caffeinated and decaffeinated.

OTHER

- Propyl gallate.

- Chlorine and chlorine by-products.

- Ethinylestradiol (combined oral contraceptive pill).

- Metalloestrogens (a class of inorganic xenoestrogens).

- Alkylphenol (surfactant used in cleaning detergents.

Final Overview

* * *

Opportunities are usually disguised as hard work, so most
people don't recognise them

– Ann Landers

S even Steps to Focus on to Begin your Journey:

Step 1- Nutritious Food & Protein Shakes

Step 2- Nutritional Supplementation

Step 3- Toxin & Xenoestrogen Removal

Step 4- Aromatase Therapy

Step 5- Hormone Therapy

Step 6- Systemic Enzyme Therapy

Step 7- Emotional Support, Counselling & Therapy

Make sure that above all else to ensure:-

- NO WHEAT, NO WHEAT, NO WHEAT, NO WHEAT, absolutely NO WHEAT

- NO SOY

- NO QUORN

- NO COFFEE

- NOTHING from the above THAT IS INFLAMMATORY
  OR INTOLERABLE FOR YOUR BODY.

Discuss with a kind and caring doctor, gynaecologist, specialist or make your own decision to:

- STOP – IUD/COILS

- STOP – BIRTH CONTROL PILL

- STOP – USING MICROWAVE

- STOP – USING PLASTIC CONTAINERS & Kettle

- STOP – PHARMACEUTICALS and DRUGS

- STOP – PAINKILLERS (if possible)

Remember to trust your instincts above all else. You know your body better than anyone else so if in doubt, check it all out.

Remember your power and rights. If you do not wish an item in your body then hold firm. Equally if you wish an item removed from your body, like a coil, again hold firm and remember that is your right to have it removed.

This is your body and you have to live in it.

Do your own wide ranging research but ultimately always trust yourself and your body over any bullying or pressurising treatment.

- TEST – HORMONE TESTS

- TEST – HAIR ANALYSIS TEST

- TEST – NUTRITIONAL DEFICIENCY/B12/FERRITIN
- TEST – DIGESTION Betaine Stomach Acid Test
- TEST – LIVER FUNCTION
- TEST – STRESS CORTISOL

- SWAP OUT – TOXIC PERSONAL PRODUCTS
- SWAP OUT – TOXIC HOUSEHOLD PRODUCTS
- SWAP OUT – TOXIC WASHING POWDERS

- EAT – 90g PROTEIN A DAY MINIMUM
- EAT – PROTEIN SHAKE
- EAT – ORGANIC FREE-RANGE FOOD
- EAT – HORMONE AND PESTICIDE-FREE
- EAT – USE THE STONE-AGE CAVEWOMAN DIET

- INTRODUCE – NUTRITIONAL SUPPLEMENTS
- INTRODUCE – NATURAL AROMATASE INHIBITORS
- INTRODUCE – NATURAL BIO-IDENTICAL PROGESTERONE
- INTRODUCE – SYSTEMIC ENZYME THERAPY
- INTRODUCE – EMOTIONAL SUPPORT

Please do not underestimate the impact of the following elements;-

TOXIC PEOPLE

Some people like family members, partners, friends, work colleagues, and associates, may be toxic. They may be mistreating you emotionally and subconsciously. Ensure that you journal and pay attention to how certain people make you feel after you have engaged with them. Do you always end up feeling 'wrong' or upset or depressed or flat or trying to make them happy but nothing does? It is an odd concept at the start to think that some people may be affecting an element of your health but once you start to increase your awareness about how you feel after an interaction with someone it may surprise you. In particular watch out for

People & Activities who are:
- Energy 'TAKING'
- Energy 'Neutral'
- Energy 'Giving'

LEARN HOW TO PUT IN BOUNDARIES WITH TOXIC PEOPLE AND LIMIT TIME SPENT WITH THEM.

You are looking to increase the number of people around you who are energy giving, kind, caring, reflective and supportive.

You will soon start to notice the difference in your emotional health to be around people that believe in you and are your cheerleaders (like our amazing EndoBoss® family!).

Lastly, consider exploring and starting the following:-

- START – DAILY RELAXATION, MINDFULNESS MEDITATION
- START – BREATHING CLASSES (check out Wim Hoff)
- START – GENTLE EXERCISE
- START – BEGINNERS YOGA
- START – JOURNALLING

And never, ever, ever give up!

FURTHER SUPPORT

Wendy wrote her book with the aim of it being able to help every woman that read it. However, Wendy realised that there are a lot of changes to take in from this book and many, many women need different degrees of support, accountability and coaching on their healing journey.

As such, Wendy created the successful 22 weeks online 'EndoBoss® Academy' online training program that works in a safe, structured and step by step fashion, addressing the root causes of inflammation and providing women with weekly support and personalised coaching from trained EndoBoss® Practitioner Coaches and herself.

After helping many women successfully complete her EndoBoss® Academy, Wendy then became aware of the even greater importance of embracing emotions on this journey as well.

This lead her to develop two further online programs on the EndoBoss® Pathway: **'Embracing Emotions, Empathy & Energy'**, and the **'Advanced Plus'** program which proceeds the **'EndoBoss® Academy'**.

Finally, Wendy, in her endeavour to help as many women out of pain as possible, has created a number of online courses of different price brackets, like the **'Unstoppable EndoBoss® 21 Day Challenge'** and also the **'EndoBoss® Practitioner Coach Training'** program.

The **'EndoBoss Practitioner Coach Training'** program helps women become Endometriosis Health Coach and pay forward their own successful journey to help others out of suffering and pain.
To learn more go to: https://HealEndometriosisNaturallyCourse.com

RESOURCES PAGE

To help you begin your new journey, Wendy has created an online page which lists some of the products, supplements, and books that she uses.

Go to https://healendometriosisnaturally.com/Resources where you find a full list of supportive resources to help you start and continue this new journey.

Also, to help you jumpstart your journey, you can download your FREE **'Top 5 Quick-Start Tips'** report at: https://HealEndometriosisNaturally.com

FINAL MESSAGE TO READER

Every kind and positive review about this book could potentially save a woman's life.

If a woman has felt rejected and failed by the medical system that she had pinned all her hopes on, hearing about how this book has helped you could give her the gift of hope and a pathway.

So, please share your positive views of your reading experience and how the content of this book has helped you – either by contacting us, or by posting a review on Amazon.

If you have left a review already online with Amazon then please email it through to us for a chance to be entered into a prize draw for a signed copy of Wendy's paperback book *Heal Endometriosis Naturally Cookbook with 101 Recipes*.

If after a few months of following the steps in this book you have noticed physical changes and want to tell us about your incredible story, then we would love to hear from you. Please share by sending with us at <u>Support@HealEndometriosisNaturally.ZohoDesk.com</u>.

You may be lucky enough to be invited as a special guest on to Wendy's 'Heal Endometriosis Naturally Podcast' and maybe even feature in the next **'Endometriosis Success Stories'** paperback book series.

ABOUT THE AUTHOR

Wendy K Laidlaw lives in Edinburgh, Scotland, with her two children, her chocolate Labrador and two cats.

Wendy is an author and endometriosis health pioneer, mentor coach, and, of course, founder of Heal Endometriosis Naturally. She hosts the podcast: 'Heal Endometriosis Naturally with Wendy K Laidlaw'. She is a business coach helping young entrepreneurs fast-track their purpose and pathway at the earliest stages of creating their online businesses.

As well as a published author, Wendy has pioneered several online programs to support women with endometriosis, adenomyosis, cysts, fibroids, and improve their infertility like;
EndoBoss® 21 Day Unstoppable EndoBoss® Challenge
Embracing Emotions, Empathy & Energy 5 Weeks Online Program
EndoBoss® Academy 22 Weeks Online Program
EndoBoss® Advanced Plus 5 Weeks Online Program,
EndoBoss® Alumni Mastery 12 Months Program
EndoBoss® Practitioner Coach Training 6 Months Program

Women who are accepted into her EndoBoss® Academy may be able to work their way through the full healing pathway and then apply to train as an EndoBoss® Practitioner Coach.

All women who complete the EndoBoss® Academy are granted the coveted title of an EndoBoss® Alumni.

All women who successfully put their condition into remission are gifted a specially commissioned **EndoBoss® Medal** to honour the battle they fought against endometriosis – and won!

Every woman with endometriosis deserves to be awarded a medal of honour and strength for what she had achieved and the decades of suffering and everything else she has gone through!

Wendy's dream is to run the world's leading training organisation for EndoBoss® Practitioner Coaches. This will then allow the training of other women, to help spread her success story and message to millions with endometriosis globally – and she hopes, that one day you will join her.

NOTES

1. Rogers, P. A. W., T. M. D'Hooghe, A. Fazleabas, C. E. Gargett, L. C. Giudice, G. W. Montgomery, L. Rombauts, L. A. Salamonsen, and K. T. Zondervan. 2009. "Priorities for Endometriosis Research: Recommendations from an International Consensus Workshop." *Reproductive Sciences* 16 (4): 335-346.

2. Zondervan, K. T., C. M. Becker, and S. A. Missmer. 2020. "Endometriosis." *The New England Journal of Medicine* 382 (1): 1244-1256.

3. Arruda, M. S., C. A. Petta, M. S. Abrão, and C. L. Benetti-Pinto. 2003. "Time Elapsed from Onset of Symptoms to Diagnosis of Endometriosis in a Cohort Study of Brazilian Women." *Human Reproduction* 18 (4): 756-759.; Endometriosis UK. 2020. *Endometriois UK.* Accessed August 5, 2020. https://www.endometriosis-uk.org/endometriosis-facts-and-figures.

4. Rier, S. E., D. C. Martin, R. E. Bowman, W. P. Dmowski, and J. L. Becker. 1993. "Endometriosis in Rhesus Monkeys (Macaca mulatta) Following Chronic Exposure to 2,3,7,8-tetrachlorodibenzo-p-dioxin." *Fundamental and Applied Toxicology* 21 (4): 433-441.

5. Bulletti, C., M. E. Coccia, S. Battistoni, and A. Borini. 2010. "Endometriosis and Infertility." *Journal of Assisted Reproduction and Genetics* 27 (8): 441-447.

6. Tommy's. 2017. *Tommy's.* September 4. Accessed July 28, 2020. https://www.tommys.org/pregnancy-information/planning-pregnancy/fertility-and-infertility/how-does-endometriosis-affect-fertility.

7. Mills, D. S., and M. Vernon. 2002. "Digestion and the Reproductive System." In *Endometriosis: A Key to Healing Through Nutrition*, 206. London: Thorsons.

8. Aitken, M., M. Kleinrock, A. Simorellis, and D. Nass. 2019. "The Global Use of Medicine in 2019 and Outlook to 2023: Forecasts and Area to Watch." *IQVIA Institute for Human Data Science.* January. Accessed July 30, 2020. https://www.iqvia.com/-/media/iqvia/pdfs/institute-reports/the-global-use-of-medicine-in-2019-and-outlook-to-2023.pdf?_=1597947756032

9. Masters, R. C., A. D. Liese, S. M. Haffner, L. E. Wagenknecht, and A. J. Hanley. 2010. "Whole and Refined Grain Intakes are Related to Inflammatory Protein Concentrations in Human Plasma." *The Journal of Nutrition* 140 (3): 587-594.

10. Gobbetti, M., C. G. Rizzello, R. D. Cagno, and M. D. Angelis. 2007. "Sourdough Lactobacilli and Celiac Disease." *International Journal of Food Microbiology* 24 (2): 187-196.

11. Belderok, B. 2000. "Developments in Bread-Making Processes." *Plant Foods for Human Nutrition* 55 (1): 1-86.

12. Singh, P., A. Arora, T. A. Strand, D. A. Leffler, C. Catassi, P. H. Green, C. P. Kelly, V. Ahuja, and G. K. Makharia. 2018. "Global Prevalence of Celiac Disease: Systematic Review and Meta-analysis." *Clinical Gastroenterology and Hepatology* 16 (1): 823-836.; Molina-Infante, J., S. Santolaria, D. S. Sanders, and F. Fernández-Bañares. 2015. "Systematic Review: Noncoeliac Gluten Sensitivity." *Alimentary Pharmacology and Therapeutics* 41 (9): 807-820.

13. Biesiekierski, J. R. 2017. "What is Gluten?" *Journal of Gastroenterology and Hepatology* 32 (S1): 78-81.

14. Ji, S. 2019. "Wheat Germ Lectin: Opening Pandora's Bread Box." *Journal of Gluten Sensitivity* 9 (1): N/A.

15. Huebner, F. R., K. W. Lieberman, R. P. Rubino, and J. S. Wall. 1984. "Demonstration of High Opioid-Like Activity in Isolated Peptides from Wheat Gluten Hydrolysates." *Peptides* 5 (6): 1139-1147.

16. Associated Press. 2016. *STAT.* September 20. Accessed August 3, 2020. https://www.statnews.com/2016/09/20/sugar-consumption-americans/.; Jeavans, C. 2014. *BBC.* June 26. Accessed August 3, 2020. https://www.bbc.co.uk/news/health-27941325.

17. DiNicolantonio, J. J., J. H. O'Keefe, and S. C. Lucan. 2015. "Added Fructose: A Principal Driver of Type 2 Diabetes Mellitus and Its Consequences." *Mayo Clinic Proceedings* 90 (3): 372-381.

18. Strickler, H. 2016. *New York Presbyterian*. Accessed August 4, 2020. https://www.nyp.org/cancer/cancerprevention/cancer-prevention-articles/026-the-relationship-between-insulin-and-cancer.

19. Yang, C. Z., S. I. Yaniger, V. C. Jordan, D. J. Klein, and G. D. Bittner. 2011. "Most Plastic Products Release Estrogenic Chemicals: A Potential Health Problem That Can Be Solved." *Environmental Health Perspectives* 119 (7): 989-996.

20. Bennett, J. M., C. P. Fagundes, and J. Kiecolt-Glaser. 2013. "The Chronic Stress of Caregiving Accelerates the Natural Aging of the Immune System." *Immunosenescence: Psychological and Behavioural Determinants* (Springer-Verlag) 1: 35-46.

21. Siegel, E. R., C. McFadden, K. Monahan, A. W. Lehren, and P. Siniauer. 2018. *NBC*. December 19. Accessed August 5, 2020. https://www.nbcnews.com/health/health-news/da-vinci-surgical-robot-medical-breakthrough-risks-patients-n949341.

22. Keshavarz, H., B. A. Kieke S. D. Hillis, and P. A. Marchbanks. 2002. "Hysterectomy Surveillance – United States, 1994-1999." *Morbidity and Mortality Weekly Report* 51 (SS05): 1-8.

23. HERS Foundation. 2018. "Adverse Effects Data." *HERS Foundation.* Accessed August 2, 2020. https://www.hersfoundation.org/adverse-effects-data/.

24. Laughlin-Tommaso, S. K., Z. Khan, A. L. Weaver, C. Y. Smith, W. A. Rocca, and E. A. Stewart. 2018. "Cardiovascular and Metabolic Morbidity After Hysterectomy with Ovarian Conservation: a Cohort Study." *Menopause* 25 (5): 483-492.

25. Parker, W. H., D. Feskanich, M. S. Broder, E. Chang, D. Shoupe, C. M. Farquhar, J. S. Berek, and J. E. Manson. 2013. "Long-term Mortality Associated with Oophorectomy versus Ovarian Conservation in the Nurses 'Health Study." *Obstetrics & Gynecology* 121 (4): 709-716.

26. Moorman, P. G., E. R. Myers, J. M. Schildkraut, E. S. Iversen, F. Wang, and N. Warren. 2011. "Effect of Hysterectomy With Ovarian Preservation on Ovarian Function." *Obstetrics & Gynecology* 118 (6): 1271-1279.

27. Carlsen, E., A. Giwercman, N. Keiding, and N. E. Skakkebaek. 1992. "Evidence for Decreasing Quality of Semen During Past 50 Years." *The British Medical Journal* 305 (6854): 609-613.

28. Vajda, A. M., L.B. Barber, J. L. Gray, E. M. Lopez, J. D. Woodling, and D. O. Norris. 2008. "Reproductive Disruption in Fish Downstream from an Estrogenic Wastewater Effluent." *Environmental Science & Technology* 42 (9): 3407-3414.

29. Richard, S., S. Moslemi, H. Sipahutar, N. Benachour, and G.-E. Seralini. 2005. "Differential Effects of Glyphosate and Roundup on Human Placental Cells and Aromatase." *Environmental Health Perspectives* 113 (6): 716-720.

30. Canadian Biotechnology Advisory Committee. 2002. "Improving the Regulation of Genetically Modified Foods and Other Novel Foods in Canada." *Government of Canada Publications.* August. Accessed August 3, 2020. http://publications.gc.ca/collections/Collection/C2-589-2001-1E.pdf.

31. Sisti, J. S., S. E. Hankinson, N. E. Caporaso, F. Gu, R. M. Tamimi, B. Rosner, X. Xu, R. Ziegler, and A. H. Eliassen. 2015. "Caffeine, Coffee and Tea Intake and Urinary

Estrogens and Estrogen Metabolites in Premenopausal Women." *Cancer Epidemiology, Biomarkers & Prevention* 24 (8): 1174-1183.

32. Breast Cancer Options. N/A. "What You Can Do To Reduce Your Exposure To Chemicals." *Breast Cancer Options.* Accessed August 8, 2020. http://breastcanceroptions.org/WHAT%20YOU%20CAN%20DO%20TO%20REDUCE%20YOUR%20EXPOSURE%20TO%20CHEMICALS.pdf.

33. FDA. December. "Ogen: estropipate tablets, USP." *USA Food & Drug Administration.* 2004. Accessed August 5, 2020.

34. Asi, N., K. Mohammed, Q. Haydour, M. R. Gionfriddo, O. L. M. Vargas, L. J. Prokop, S. S. Faubion, and M. H. Murad. 2016. "Progesterone vs. Synthetic Progestins and the Risk of Breast Cancer: A Systematic Review and Meta-Analysis." *Systematic Reviews* 5 (1): 121.

35. Guerrero, C. A. H., L. B. Montenegro, J. J. Díaz, J. M. Cabrera, and P. B. Valencia. 2006. "Endometriosis and Deficient Intake of Antioxidants Molecules Related to Peripheral and Peritoneal Oxidative Stress." *Ginecología y Obstetricia de México* 74 (1): 20-28.

36. Esch, P. M., H. Gerngross, and A. Fabian. 1989. "Reduction of Postoperative Swelling: Objective Measurement of Swelling of the Upper Ankle Joint in Treatment with Serrapeptase." *Fortschritte der Medizin* 107 (4): 67-8, 71-2.

37. Harvard Healthbeat. 2020. "Writing About Emotions May Ease Stress and Trauma." *Harvard Health Publishing: Harvard Medical School.* Accessed August 7, 2020. https://www.health.harvard.edu/healthbeat/writing-about-emotions-may-ease-stress-and-trauma.

38. Shapero, B. G., J. Greenberg, P. Pedrelli, M. d. Jong, and G. Desbordes. 2018. "Mindfulness-Based Interventions in Psychiatry." *FOCUS: The Journal of Lifelong Learning in Psychiatry* 16 (1): 32-39.

BIBLIOGRAPHY

Aitken, M., M. Kleinrock, A. Simorellis, and D. Nass. 2019. "The Global Use of Medicine in 2019 and Outlook to 2023: Forecasts and Area to Watch." *IQVIA Institute for Human Data Science.* January. Accessed July 30, 2020. https://www.iqvia.com/-/media/iqvia/pdfs/institute-reports/the-global-use-of-medicine-in-2019-and-outlook-to-2023.pdf?_=1597947756032.

Arruda, M. S., C. A. Petta, M. S. Abrão, and C. L. Benetti-Pinto. 2003. "Time Elapsed from Onset of Symptoms to Diagnosis of Endometriosis in a Cohort Study of Brazilian Women." *Human Reproduction* 18 (4): 756-759.

Asi, N., K. Mohammed, Q. Haydour, M. R. Gionfriddo, O. L. M. Vargas, L. J. Prokop, S. S. Faubion, and M. H. Murad. 2016. "Progesterone vs. Synthetic Progestins and the Risk of Breast Cancer: A Systematic Review and Meta-Analysis." *Systematic Reviews* 5 (1): 121.

Associated Press. 2016. *STAT.* September 20. Accessed August 3, 2020. https://www.statnews.com/2016/09/20/sugar-consumption-americans/.

Belderok, B. 2000. "Developments in Bread-Making Processes." *Plant Foods for Human Nutrition* 55 (1): 1-86.

Bennett, J. M., C. P. Fagundes, and J. Kiecolt-Glaser. 2013. "The Chronic Stress of Caregiving Accelerates the Natural Aging of the Immune System." *Immunosenescence: Psychological and Behavioural Determinants* (Springer-Verlag) 1: 35-46.

Biesiekierski, J. R. 2017. "What is Gluten?" *Journal of Gastroenterology and Hepatology* 32 (S1): 78-81.

Breast Cancer Options. N/A. "What You Can Do To Reduce Your Exposure To Chemicals." *Breast Cancer Options.* Accessed August 8, 2020. http://breastcanceroptions.org/WHAT%20YOU%20CAN%20DO%20TO%20REDUCE%20YOUR%20EXPOSURE%20TO%20CHEMICALS.pdf.

Bulletti, C., M. E. Coccia, S. Battistoni, and A. Borini. 2010. "Endometriosis and Infertility." *Journal of Assisted Reproduction and Genetics* 27 (8): 441-447.

Canadian Biotechnology Advisory Committee. 2002. "Improving the Regulation of Genetically Modified Foods and Other Novel Foods in Canada." *Government of Canada Publications.* August. Accessed August 3, 2020. http://publications.gc.ca/collections/Collection/C2-589-2001-1E.pdf.

Carlsen, E., A. Giwercman, N. Keiding, and N. E. Skakkebaek. 1992. "Evidence for Decreasing Quality of Semen During Past 50 Years." *The British Medical Journal* 305 (6854): 609-613.

DiNicolantonio, J. J., J. H. O'Keefe, and S. C. Lucan. 2015. "Added Fructose: A Principal Driver of Type 2 Diabetes Mellitus and Its Consequences." *Mayo Clinic Proceedings* 90 (3): 372-381.

Endometriosis UK. 2020. *Endometriois UK.* Accessed August 5, 2020. https://www.endometriosis-uk.org/endometriosis-facts-and-figures.

Esch, P. M., H. Gerngross, and A. Fabian. 1989. "Reduction of Postoperative Swelling: Objective Measurement of Swelling of the Upper Ankle Joint in Treatment with Serrapeptase." *Fortschritte der Medizin* 107 (4): 67-8, 71-2.

FDA. December. "Ogen: estropipate tablets, USP." *USA Food & Drug Administration.* 2004. Accessed August 5, 2020. https://www.accessdata.fda.gov/drugsatfda_docs/label/2005/083220s041lbl.pdf.

Gobbetti, M., C. G. Rizzello, R. D. Cagno, and M. D. Angelis. 2007. "Sourdough Lactobacilli and Celiac Disease." *International Journal of Food Microbiology* 24 (2): 187-196.

Guerrero, C. A. H., L. B. Montenegro, J. J. Díaz, J. M. Cabrera, and P. B. Valencia. 2006. "Endometriosis and Deficient Intake of Antioxidants Molecules Related to Peripheral and Peritoneal Oxidative Stress." *Ginecología y Obstetricia de México* 74 (1): 20-28.

Harvard Healthbeat. 2020. "Writing About Emotions May Ease Stress and Trauma." *Harvard Health Publishing: Harvard Medical School.* Accessed August 7, 2020. https://www.health.harvard.edu/healthbeat/writing-about-emotions-may-ease-stress-and-trauma.

HERS Foundation. 2018. "Adverse Effects Data." *HERS Foundation.* Accessed August 2, 2020. https://www.hersfoundation.org/adverse-effects-data/.

Huebner, F. R., K. W. Lieberman, R. P. Rubino, and J. S. Wall. 1984. "Demonstration of High Opioid-Like Activity in Isolated Peptides from Wheat Gluten Hydrolysates." *Peptides* 5 (6): 1139-1147.

Jeavans, C. 2014. *BBC.* June 26. Accessed August 3, 2020. https://www.bbc.co.uk/news/health-27941325.

Ji, S. 2019. "Wheat Germ Lectin: Opening Pandora's Bread Box." *Journal of Gluten Sensitivity* 9 (1): N/A.

Keshavarz, H., B. A. Kieke S. D. Hillis, and P. A. Marchbanks. 2002. "Hysterectomy Surveillance – United States, 1994-1999." *Morbidity and Mortality Weekly Report* 51 (SS05): 1-8.

Laughlin-Tommaso, S. K., Z. Khan, A. L. Weaver, C. Y. Smith, W. A. Rocca, and E. A. Stewart. 2018. "Cardiovascular and Metabolic Morbidity After Hysterectomy with Ovarian Conservation: A Cohort Study." *Menopause* 25 (5): 483-492.

Masters, R. C., A. D. Liese, S. M. Haffner, L. E. Wagenknecht, and A. J. Hanley. 2010. "Whole and Refined Grain Intakes are Related to Inflammatory Protein Concentrations in Human Plasma." *The Journal of Nutrition* 140 (3): 587-594.

Mills, D. S., and M. Vernon. 2002. "Digestion and the Reproductive System." In *Endometriosis: A Key to Healing Through Nutrition*, 206. London: Thorsons.

Molina-Infante, J., S. Santolaria, D. S. Sanders, and F. Fernández-Bañares. 2015. "Systematic Review: Noncoeliac Gluten Sensitivity." *Alimentary Pharmacology and Therapeutics* 41 (9): 807-820.

Moorman, P. G., E. R. Myers, J. M. Schildkraut, E. S. Iversen, F. Wang, and N. Warren. 2011. "Effect of Hysterectomy With Ovarian Preservation on Ovarian Function." *Obstetrics & Gynecology* 118 (6): 1271-1279.

Parker, W. H., D. Feskanich, M. S. Broder, E. Chang, D. Shoupe, C. M. Farquhar, J. S. Berek, and J. E. Manson. 2013. "Long-term Mortality Associated with Oophorectomy versus Ovarian Conservation in the Nurses 'Health Study." *Obstetrics & Gynecology* 121 (4): 709-716.

Richard, S., S. Moslemi, H. Sipahutar, N. Benachour, and G.-E. Seralini. 2005. "Differential Effects of Glyphosate and Roundup on Human Placental Cells and Aromatase." *Environmental Health Perspectives* 113 (6): 716-720.

Rier, S. E., D. C. Martin, R. E. Bowman, W. P. Dmowski, and J. L. Becker. 1993. "Endometriosis in Rhesus Monkeys (Macaca mulatta) Following Chronic Exposure to 2,3,7,8-tetrachlorodibenzo-p-dioxin." *Fundamental and Applied Toxicology* 21 (4): 433-441.

Rogers, P. A. W., T. M. D'Hooghe, A. Fazleabas, C. E. Gargett, L. C. Giudice, G. W. Montgomery, L. Rombauts, L. A. Salamonsen, and K. T. Zondervan. 2009. "Priorities for Endometriosis Research: Recommendations from an International Consensus Workshop." *Reproductive Sciences* 16 (4): 335-346.

Shapero, B. G., J. Greenberg, P. Pedrelli, M. d. Jong, and G. Desbordes. 2018. "Mindfulness-Based Interventions in Psychiatry." *FOCUS: The Journal of Lifelong Learning in Psychiatry* 16 (1): 32-39.

Siegel, E. R., C. McFadden, K. Monahan, A. W. Lehren, and P. Siniauer. 2018. *NBC*.
    December 19. Accessed August 5, 2020.
    https://www.nbcnews.com/health/health-news/da-vinci-surgical-robot-medical-
    breakthrough-risks-patients-n949341.

Singh, P., A. Arora, T. A. Strand, D. A. Leffler, C. Catassi, P. H. Green, C. P. Kelly, V.
    Ahuja, and G. K. Makharia. 2018. "Global Prevalence of Celiac Disease:
    Systematic Review and Meta-analysis." *Clinical Gastroenterology and Hepatology* 16 (1):
    823-836.

Sisti, J. S., S. E. Hankinson, N. E. Caporaso, F. Gu, R. M. Tamimi, B. Rosner, X. Xu, R.
    Ziegler, and A. H. Eliassen. 2015. "Caffeine, Coffee and Tea Intake and Urinary
    Estrogens and Estrogen Metabolites in Premenopausal Women." *Cancer
    Epidemiology, Biomarkers & Prevention* 24 (8): 1174-1183.

Strickler, H. 2016. *New York Presbyterian* . Accessed August 4, 2020.
    https://www.nyp.org/cancer/cancerprevention/cancer-prevention-articles/026-
    the-relationship-between-insulin-and-cancer.

Tommy's. 2017. *Tommy's*. September 4. Accessed July 28, 2020.
    https://www.tommys.org/pregnancy-information/planning-pregnancy/fertility-
    and-infertility/how-does-endometriosis-affect-fertility.

Vajda, A. M., L.B. Barber, J. L. Gray, E. M. Lopez, J. D. Woodling, and D. O. Norris. 2008.
    "Reproductive Disruption in Fish Downstream from an Estrogenic Wastewater
    Effluent." *Environmental Science & Technology* 42 (9): 3407-3414.

Yang, C. Z., S. I. Yaniger, V. C. Jordan, D. J. Klein, and G. D. Bittner. 2011. "Most Plastic
    Products Release Estrogenic Chemicals: A Potential Health Problem That Can Be
    Solved." *Environmental Health Perspectives* 119 (7): 989-996.

Zondervan, K. T., C. M. Becker, and S. A. Missmer. 2020. "Endometriosis." *The New England
    Journal of Medicine* 382 (1): 1244-1256.

How I Ended My Endometriosis Naturally

And now it's your turn to end yours!

Made in the USA
Middletown, DE
28 April 2022

64870247R00156